D0291109

"INSPIRING . . . ENCOURAGING . . . TENDERLY AND COMPASSIONATELY WRITTEN, IT ACTS ALMOST LIKE A LOVING COMPANION." —*Modern Maturity*

What kind of life would you be living if you adjusted the world to yourself instead of—as most patients generally have done— adjusting yourself to the world? What kind of life and lifestyle would make you glad to get up in the morning and glad to go to bed at night?

These are the questions Dr. LeShan asks of his patients in order to open their eyes to the "turning point" that can make the difference in their lives—and their cancer treatment. His methods get impressive results—over the past 30 years, approximately half of his patients with poor prognoses have experienced long-term remission and are still alive. Nearly all dramatically improved their emotional state and quality of life.

"CANCER AS A TURNING POINT is the summation by a great pioneer of cancer psychotherapy of his creative, original, and iconoclastic contribution to the field."
—*Advances*

"INSPIRING." —*Library Journal*

LAWRENCE LESHAN, Ph.D., has been a research and clinical psychologist for more than forty-five years. A graduate of William and Mary, he is the author of over a dozen books, including *You Can Fight for Your Life: Emotional Factors in the Treatment of Cancer* and *The Mechanic and the Gardener: How to Use the Holistic Revolution in Medicine.*

ALSO BY LAWRENCE LeSHAN

LAWRENCE LeSHAN, Ph.D.

CANCER AS A TURNING POINT

*A Handbook for People
with Cancer, Their Families,
and Health Professionals*

Ⓟ
A PLUME BOOK

PLUME

Published by the Penguin Group

Penguin Books USA Inc., 375 Hudson Street, New York, New York 10014, U.S.A.

Penguin Books Ltd, 27 Wrights Lane, London W8 5TZ, England

Penguin Books Australia Ltd, Ringwood, Victoria, Australia

Penguin Books Canada Ltd, 2801 John Street, Markham, Ontario, Canada L3R 1B4

Penguin Books (N.Z.) Ltd, 182-190 Wairau Road, Auckland 10, New Zealand

Penguin Books Ltd, Registered Offices: Harmondsworth, Middlesex, England

Cancer as a Turning Point was previously published in a Dutton edition, and published simultaneously in Canada by Fitzhenry & Whiteside Limited.

First Plume Printing, May 1990

10 9 8 7 6 5 4 3 2 1

Grateful acknowledgment is given for permission to quote from the following works:

"Adelaide's Lament" by Frank Loesser from Guys and Dolls *copyright © 1950 by Frank Music Corp. Copyright renewed © 1978 by Frank Music Corp. International copyright secured. All rights reserved. Used by permission.*

Brian Inglis, The Case for Unorthodox Medicine *(New York: Putnam, 1967), pp. 43–44. Copyright © 1967 by Brian Inglis. Reproduced by kind permission of Curtis Brown, London.*

LIBRARY OF CONGRESS CATALOGING-IN-PUBLICATION DATA

LeShan, Lawrence L., 1920-

    Cancer as a turning point : a handbook for people with cancer, their families, and health professionals / Lawrence LeShan.

       p.   cm.

    Reprint. Originally published: New York : Dutton, c1989.

    Includes bibliographical references.

    ISBN 0-452-26419-7

    1. Cancer—Psychosomatic aspects. 2. Holistic medicine.

I. Title.

    [DNLM: 1. Holistic Health—popular works. 2.Neoplasms—psychology—popular works. 3. Neoplasms—therapy—popular works.

QZ 201 L629c 1989a]

RC262.L37   1990

616.99'406—dc20

DNLM/DLC

for Library of Congress   90-5596
                                                CIP

 REGISTERED TRADEMARK—MARCA REGISTRADA

Printed in the United States of America

Original hardcover book designed by Steven N. Stathakis

A Note to the Reader: *The ideas, procedures, and suggestions contained in this book are not intended as a substitute for consulting with your physician. All matters regarding your health require medical supervision.*

This book is dedicated with love, respect, and gratitude to my daughter Wendy. All during her early childhood she was too often denied the attention she needed from a father who was constantly struggling to understand and help patients with catastrophic illnesses. When, after fifteen years, I decided to begin a different research project, she was outraged. She told me it was immoral not to continue to help people with cancer after I had made some progress. I had to promise her I would not abandon patients who sought my help, no matter what else I might be working on. I have never been more proud of anyone because she had paid a heavy price for my work.

ACKNOWLEDGMENTS

I wish to express my deep gratitude to Frederick Ayer II for his long support of this work. Without him this book would not have been possible. I owe a profound debt to the people with cancer who taught me all that I know over these last thirty-five years. My appreciation also to the increasing number of therapists all over the world who are using this approach.

I'd also like to pay tribute to my wife, Eda LeShan, who shared the joys and pains of this adventure and whose contributions to this book are very great.

CONTENTS

CONTENTS

PREFACE

Those closely involved with cancer—patients, families, friends, health professionals—very rarely have information in one crucial area: how to mobilize the patient's self-healing abilities and bring them to the aid of the medical program.

This state-of-the-art handbook gathers, for the first time in one place, the known information on this subject. The book comes out of a thirty-five-year research project involving several thousand people with cancer. It is designed to teach those with the illness and their families, friends, physicians, clergymen, and psychotherapists how to use psychological change to help heal the patient's compromised immune system.

I believe a serious problem has arisen in recent years. Despite professional background in associated areas, some individuals have a very limited knowledge of the field and have interpreted this approach as one that blames the patient for the illness. They say that in addition to the anxiety and pain of cancer, a new guilt has been added—guilt arising from a false idea, guilt that is an intolerable load for the patient.

These critics talk complete nonsense. *Thoughts and feelings do not cause cancer and cannot cure cancer.* But they are one factor, and an important one, in the total ecology that makes up a human being. Feelings affect body chemistry (which affects the development or regression of a tumor), just as body chemistry affects feelings. The emerging science related to the nature of the immune system has merely reinforced the belief that certain kinds of stress lower the ability of the body's chemistry to withstand disease. There is, as William James once remarked, no clear dividing line between a person's philosophy and physiology, between mind and body. All the different aspects of a person interact with, and influence, each other.

What we have learned is that the immune system is strongly affected by feelings, and that taking certain kinds of psychological action can affect the immune system positively. Sometimes this makes a crucial difference in how well the medical program works. To put it in other words, there are certain psychological steps people with cancer can take to increase their self-healing and self-repair abilities and bring these more strongly to the aid of the medical program. Whether or not this will make a crucial difference in a patient's return to health depends on the total situation, including such factors as genetic endowment and the life experiences the person has had since birth.

In this approach, the patient is *not* blamed in any way for the cancer. Anyone who even hints that the person with cancer is responsible for getting it and/or for not getting better is not only the rankest amateur and should be completely ignored, but is setting in motion confusion, anxiety, and anger at the self. And those who hint that this approach increases the guilt of the patient simply do not know what they are talking about.

While there is still much to learn about the subject, we do know one additional fact: the same psychological approach that leads to the fullest effectiveness of the immune system is the approach that leads to the fullest and richest life—both during the time a person has cancer and afterward.

The form of this book has been strongly influenced by my experience in five or six dozen seminars on the subject that I have given over the past twenty years. These were from one to three days in length, and each included fifty to one hundred participants. For the first five years I did two kinds of seminars:

one for cancer patients and their families, and the other for health professionals. Then, by mistake, a seminar notice was poorly worded and the group that showed up was half patients and family members and half health professionals working in the cancer field. I found this out ten minutes before the meeting started. My anxiety level hit record heights! Not knowing what else to do, I announced to the group that part of the time I planned to work with them as if they were all people with cancer and the rest of the time as if they were all professionals in the field. For all concerned, the seminar was the best and most exciting that I had ever given.

Since then, I have used this format wherever possible and, judging by the reactions of the people involved, it has been highly successful. Because of this rewarding experience in "mixed seminars," I decided the only way to write this book was for a mixed audience as well.

You will find that in any specific section of this book, I may be more directly addressing the patient, the family member, or the professional. This is deliberate. We do not live in a vacuum. The heart of the modern holistic approach is that *all* levels of a person's being, their physical, psychological, spiritual aspects, their relationships and their environment, are important and none can be ignored without peril. It is only by approaching the problem of cancer from the viewpoint of the person who has the illness, of the family, and of the health professional that we can see how to best mobilize the healing and self-healing resources available so that the medical program can be most fully effective.

This is not mere speculation. Over and over again I have seen one of two things happen when the total environment of the person with cancer is mobilized for life and his or her inner ecology is thereby changed in a positive way. For some, the patient's life is prolonged, not in an arbitrary way, but in order that that there may be more experience of the self, self-recognition and the recognition—and often fulfillment—of dreams. And then there were the genuine miracles—not magic, but dedicated devotion and hard work which made the cancer a turning point in the person's life rather than a sign of its ending.

The more we learn about human biology and psychology, the more we learn about how to change and improve the *quality* and *ambiance* of life both internal and external, the more this second result may become commonplace. That surely is the hope of this book.

CANCER AS A TURNING POINT

THIRTY–FIVE YEARS OF MIND–BODY CANCER RESEARCH

. . . let me speak to you regarding the things of which you must most beware. To get angry and shout at times pleases me, for this will keep up your natural heat; but what displeases me is your being grieved and taking all matters to heart. For it is this, as the whole of physic teaches, which destroys our body more than any other cause.

Letter written by MAESTRO
LORENZO SASSOLI, *a physician, to a*
patient in 1402*

Maria was a Brazilian physician who loved her work as a pediatrician. Her husband was an electrical engineer who wanted only to be a poet. He hated his field of work, at which he was actually quite successful professionally. Their twin daughters, aged fifteen and a half when I first saw Maria, were apparently of very high artistic caliber. Both wanted to be actresses and had already had minor parts on the stage in small theaters.

*Quoted in Iris Origo, *The Merchant of Prato* (New York: Alfred A. Knopf, 1957).

When the daughters were ten, their talent was recognized by a well-known theatrical director. It crystallized Maria's decision to leave the Rio de Janeiro she loved so much and emigrate to London, where her daughters could receive the best education in the theater and where her husband could devote himself full time to his poetry. She told me she had not been "back home" since her arrival in England.

Maria could not, however, find work in London as a pediatrician that would bring in the necessary income for the needs of her family. The position she had been promised failed to materialize at the last moment.

She was offered a position with an adequate financial return in an oncology partnership, where she would deal chiefly with children and young people suffering from the childhood leukemias, Wilms' tumors, and so on. She disliked the work intensely, but continued it in order to support her husband and daughters. She also hated London and constantly missed Rio, where she had grown up. She described with enthusiasm and gusto the lovely beaches, the gentle climate, the easygoing and tolerant attitudes of the people, the striking architecture, and the friends she had had there: "I always felt *at home* wherever I was in the city. Every street felt like my own living room." She even missed speaking in her own language, she told me rather shyly.

At the age of forty-eight, she noticed a lump in her breast. She did nothing about this for over a year. By the time she had it examined by a professional colleague, it had grown several times larger. The diagnosis was adenocarcinoma of the breast. In her and her colleague's opinion, the metastases were too widespread for surgery to be an option. A course of chemotherapy was decided on, but everyone agreed that the prognosis was very poor.

I was speaking at her hospital in London during this period, and afterward she asked me for a professional appointment. We talked for an hour about her history and about her hopes and fears for the future. She saw no possibility of work that she would enjoy, of living where she would like to, or of a life that would make her glad and excited to get out of bed in the morning. Her husband and her children were very happy with their lives and she was successful enough to enable them to continue it. Rather brutally, because I felt I had to shock her into taking some action on her own behalf, I asked her how she planned to continue supporting them in the style to which they had grown accustomed after she was in the cemetery, as her cancer prognosis was so poor. She looked completed defeated. After a long pause she said: "I know I can't do it anymore. I had hoped that you would know a road for me." Her sadness and despair moved me deeply, and for a few minutes we both just sat there.

I then said that I could see no reason for her body to work hard to save her life, no reason for it to mobilize her immune system and bring its resources to the aid of the chemotherapy. By her actions, she was telling her body that it was always someone else's turn and never hers. Everyone else would be taken care of except her. Clearly she was telling herself that she was not worth fighting for. She listened, thought a bit, and then said, "It's sort of as if I keep telling myself that *for me* it's always jam yesterday and jam tomorrow, but never jam today." We agreed about this message and sat in sad and companionable silence for a while.

It was clearly an emergency situation. She was in very bad shape both physically and emotionally and clearly going down-hill on both levels. There was little to lose. I would be leaving London in a few days and I have never been very good working over the telephone or by mail. The philosopher and spiritual leader Edgar Jackson has pointed out that in some situations, the careful man is only a short step away from the paltry man. I told Maria the story of the woman who was sunbathing nude. A lovely chickadee flew down and perched on her ankle. She smiled lovingly at it. Then a great orange-and-black butterfly alighted on her knee. Again she smiled warmly. A magnificent dragonfly with its iridescent wings settled on her shoulder. It also received her welcoming smile, as did a beautiful goldfinch that came down and perched on her toes. Then a mosquito came down, settled on her breast, and bit her. She looked at it and said, "All right. *Everybody off!*"

At the punchline, Maria laughed much harder than the joke deserved. Then she sat apparently thinking very intently for several minutes. Finally she looked at me and an impish and devilish grin spread across her face. "Do you think I *really could?*" she asked.

She was as ready for action as a tomcat with its tail up. She had only needed a direction and a trigger. I had provided the direction in my lecture, and our discussion was the trigger. It was a pleasure to watch her move. I had heard of the "fiery, tempestuous Brazilian personality" before but had never expected to see the stereotype in full bloom.

That night Maria called a family conference and announced (apparently in no uncertain terms) that it was her turn now. Changes would have to be made as she could no longer afford to support her entire family. If she died they were all on their own anyway, so they might as well all take a desperate and final chance to help her immune system come to the aid of the chemotherapy. She had, she told them, been an oncologist long enough to know that with a cancer like hers, this was the only chance. In order to help this happen, there needed to be some major changes in her and their life-styles.

First, she said, her husband: quite a number of successful poets had supported themselves by working at regular jobs. If he wanted to follow the example of his particular idol, Edwin Arlington Robinson, and work as a ticket seller in the Underground, this was fine with her, but she felt he would do better as a draftsman or something like that even though he'd been away from engineering for eight years. Then, the children: they were going to leave the special private schools they had been going to and go to regular public schools. They could continue some of their private acting lessons, but would also have to get part-time jobs if this were at all possible, and even if it weren't! Certainly they could work as salesgirls, waitresses, or whatever during summer and Christmas vacations unless they had professional employment. The maid would go and all of them would pitch in with the housework. She herself was going to give up her job, take a residency in pediatrics in order to catch up with the latest techniques, and then take it from there. Moving back to Brazil when the twins were established and on their own was left as a possibility for the future.

It must have been quite a family meeting. By the end of it everyone had agreed to the new agenda and, Maria told me, "with a lot less upset and resistance than I expected. I found that they cared for me, loved me, even if I couldn't support them anymore. I'm surprised to find out that this surprised me!"

In the next six months her husband obtained a fairly low-level job in an engineering firm. He said it demanded little of him and left him with a good deal of energy for his poetry. (He had, over the years, been reasonably successful at this—he'd published two volumes of his poems and also poems in a number of magazines. These books paid him the very small amount that books of poetry generally do.) The daughters did get part-time jobs and expressed a good deal of resentment about having to do so. They complained in typically adolescent fashion and constantly had to be reminded about their household chores. Both paid for their acting lessons and also obtained a number of small jobs making television commercials and in obscure, avant-garde theaters. Maria resigned from her oncology position and took a residency in pediatrics. After a year she began working full time in this field. She was paid far less than she had earned in oncology, but enjoyed it far more.

At my suggestion, she had also consulted a nutritionist in order to upgrade her diet and to help both to potentiate the chemotherapy treatment and to avoid the worst negative side effects.

I kept in touch with her. The chemotherapy program worked far beyond expectations. The tumor masses shrank but did not disappear. At present, four years later, the medical situation seems at least temporarily stabilized and is on a watch-and-wait basis. She feels that her life is rich and exciting. Summer vacations have been spent in Rio de Janeiro. Since money is so short she has gone by herself most of the time. They have not yet decided whether or not to move back there in the next few years.

——————— ▬ ———————

The work that led to this book began in 1947 when a psychologist friend of mine, Dr. Richard Worthington, told me that he had been looking at personality tests of several people with cancer. He felt that their emotional life history somehow played a part in the development of their illness, and that this should be investigated. Dick is the best person with these kinds of personality tests I have ever known—he has a brilliant and profound understanding of them—and I had learned never to ignore anything of this sort that he said. I tucked the idea away in the back of my mind for future exploration.

Two years later I was back in the army.* Working in a very depressing job in an army mental hygiene clinic in Arkansas, I needed something interesting to fill my mind. I went back to Dick's idea and began to examine it.

The County Medical Society had a library that had been started in the early 1800s. Since then, all the local physicians had willed their books to it. I began to go there evenings. Looking at the data with a psychologist's eye, it seemed clear that psychological factors might very well have played some part in at least a good percentage of the cancer statistics.

The higher cancer mortality rates for widows and widowers that were not related to age, occupation, reproductive accomplishment, diet, or any other obvious factor were only one example of the evidence that there was something here worth looking into.

When I again left the army two years later, I talked to Dick

*After World War II, I had answered yes when the army asked me if I would remain in the Reserves. I had the idea that this was a sort of alumni association!

about what I had found. He was impressed. He called a group of businessmen together, we both made a pitch, formed a foundation, and raised enough money to support me half time for a year. I stayed on the project full time for fourteen years and part time for another twenty-two. This book is the result of that work.

As I began to work intensively, the first thing I found was that up to 1900 the relationship between cancer and psychological factors had been commonly accepted in medical circles. I went through the major cancer textbooks of the nineteenth century (using the old rule of thumb that if it went through three editions, it qualified as a major textbook). All but one of the nineteen I found said the same thing: "Of course, the emotional life history [they used a lot of different phrases for this, but the meaning was the same] plays a major role in the tendency of the person to get cancer and in the progress of the cancer." In my 1959 review of this literature for the *Journal of the National Cancer Institute,* my problem was not to find statements of this kind but rather to select which of the many ones to quote.

What had happened was plain. Dedicated nineteenth-century physicians working with cancer patients had none of the sophisticated instruments and devices we have today. Without biochemical tests and without X rays, to say nothing of CAT scans (computerized axial tomography) and the like, they had to *listen* to their patients in order to learn what was going on. And in this listening, they heard about the patient's feelings and history. The factors of great emotional loss and of hopelessness occurring *before* the first signs of the cancer were so repetitive and frequent that they could not be ignored.

Here is not the place to review that extensive literature.* A few quotations from my article are in order, however, to give some of its flavor.

As early as 1759, Gendron stressed the importance in cancer of "Disasters in Life, as occasion much trouble and

---

*Some of these works, and some reviews of this literature, are listed in the Resource Directory.

grief." He presented a long series of cases, typical of which are the following:

> Mrs. Emerson, upon the Death of her Daughter, underwent Great Affliction, and perceived her Breast to swell, which soon after grew Painful; at last broke out in a most inveterate Cancer, which consumed a great Part of it in a short Time. She had always enjoyed a perfect state of Health.
>
> The Wife of Mate of a Ship (who was taken some Time ago by the French and put in Prison) was thereby so much affected that her Breast began to swell, and soon after broke out in a desperate Cancer which had proceeded so far that I could not undertake her case. She never before had any complaint in her Breast.

In 1802 a group of the leading physicians in England and Wales formed an organization with the optimistic and cheerful name of The Society for the Prevention and Cure of Cancer. They published a list of eleven questions, each describing an area in which they felt the need for further research. One of the questions was "Is there a predisposing temperament?"

In 1846 Walter Hoyle Walshe published his treatise *The Nature and Treatment of Cancer*. This became the definitive work of the period. He covered all that was then known about the subject. Walshe was a highly trained and respected man and ". . . apparently was conversant with all that had been written and said about cancer to his time." Walshe posed his viewpoint clearly and forcefully:

> Much has been written on the influence of mental misery, sudden reverses of fortune, and habitual gloominess of temper on the deposion of carcinomatous matter. If systematic writers can be credited, these constitute the most powerful cause of the disease; . . . although the alleged influence of mental disquietude has never been made a matter of demonstration, it would be vain to deny that facts of a very

convincing character in respect to the agency of the mind in the production of this disease are frequently observed. I have myself met with cases in which the connection appeared so clear that I have decided questioning its reality would have seemed a struggle against reason.

Walshe made certain recommendations to members of families with a history of cancer, which illustrate the strength of his belief in this viewpoint. He advised them to use great care in their choice of professions, avoiding those

. . . the active and serious exercise of which entails a more or less constant care and anxiety. The importance of this consideration appears from what I have said on the influence of mental suffering in generating the disease. For this reason, the professions of the Bar, Medicine and Diplomacy should be avoided. . . . All things considered, the professions of the Army, Navy and the Church, unless there be some special objection, offer the best chance of escape from the diseases to individuals predisposed to cancer.

By implication, Walshe was clearly stating that a genetic readiness plus a long-term psychological stress results in cancer.

In this country, Willard Parker summed up in 1885 his fifty-three years of surgical experience with cancer.

It is a fact that grief is especially associated with the disease. If cancer patients were as a rule cheerful before the malignant development made its appearance, the psychological theory, no matter how logical, must fail: but it is otherwise. The fact substantiates what reason points out.

Long before this, Sir James Paget, in his classic *Surgical Pathology,* had written:

The cases are so frequent in which deep anxiety, deferred hope and disappointment are quickly followed by the growth

and increase of cancer, that we can hardly doubt that mental depression is a weighty additive to the other influences favoring the development of the cancerous constitution.

Sir Thomas Watson in 1871, phrased his conclusion as follows:

Great mental stress has been assigned as influential in hastening the development of cancerous disease in persons already predisposed. In my long life of experience, I have so often noticed this sequence that I cannot but think the imputation is true.

Herbert Snow, working at the London Cancer Hospital, was deeply impressed by Paget's view as well as the reports of other predecessors. In three books written in 1883, 1890, and 1893, he presented in detail his research findings and his concepts. In his last book, he wrote:

We are logically impelled to inquire if the great majority of cases may not own a neurotic origin? . . . We find that the number of instances in which malignant disease of the breast and uterus follows immediately antecedent emotion of a depressing character is too large to be set down to chance, or to that general liability to the buffets of ill fortune which the cancer patients, in their passage through life, share with most other people not so afflicted.

The physicians who wrote these statements were the leading specialists of the time. Their names are even today well known in medical circles.

Thus the fact that cancer and the patient's emotional life history were linked was commonly accepted in medical circles up to 1900. At that point, this viewpoint began to disappear very rapidly from the textbooks and journals. There are a number of reasons for this. The psychosomatic viewpoint had been going more and more out of fashion for fifty years. Further, surgery that was both painless and antiseptic had been developed in the preceding fifteen years and was now making its big bid as the way to deal with cancer. Surgery focuses our attention on cancer as a local disease of a specific part of the body and not as one aspect of a total human being's functioning, which is the essence of the psychosomatic view. Radiation, coming along shortly thereafter as a therapy method, reinforced this concept of cancer as a local body problem.

Another reason for the change was that a psychosomatic theory was useless at this time. Psychiatry was barely into the descriptive phase, and there were no tools with which to explore the matter further or to use to try to intervene in the processes involved. There was simply nothing to do with the information on the mind–body relationship in cancer—no techniques available to use to make it useful.

So, gradually, the idea that cancer was related to the total life history of the person disappeared from the literature and from the currently accepted concepts in medicine. A few physicians tried to keep it alive, but to no avail. For half a century it was almost unknown.

The situation has now changed completely. Since 1955 literally dozens of studies have shown conclusively that the emotional life history often does play an important part in determining an individual's resistance to getting cancer and in how a cancer develops after it appears. It is certainly not the only factor and does not play a part for every person with cancer by a long shot, but every cancer patient's emotional life history should be considered. Further, we now have the techniques and tools to explore the matter much more deeply, and many such studies have been undertaken. These studies are both retrospective (exploring patients' emotional life history after the cancer appeared) and prospective (predicting the future from psychological factors) in nature. A good example of the predictive studies is the work of Ronald Greer and his group. Greer interviewed a number of women who had had mastectomies. On the basis of the interview (three months after the operation) he divided them into classes according to their attitudes. He then simply observed what happened to the women for over fifteen years. He found out that, as he had predicted, some classes showed a statistically significantly higher survival rate than others. For example, the "feisty" (I'm going to lick this thing and no one is going to stop me) group showed a far higher survival rate than the "apathetic" (My life is over and nothing is worthwhile any longer) group.

A great many studies are now available. A list of some of the most significant and of some reviews of this literature is presented in the Resource Directory. A recent study by David Spiegel and others reported in *The Lancet* shows that psychological treatment had a definite, positive effect on women with metasticised breast cancer.

However, at the time I started the research that led to this book, the present-day literature was skimpy indeed. There were no guidelines that could be depended on. All I knew was that there were enough strong clues to make the subject really worth investigation.

In 1952, with a research grant and enough clinical and research training to do legitimate work, I applied to the leading hospitals in New York City. I fully expected to have no difficulty in finding a place to work, since the purpose of the grant was simply to investigate the fruitfulness of looking at cancer as a disease whose presence and development were influenced by personality factors. To my surprise, the first fifteen hospitals I applied to turned me down, sometimes with shocking rapidity. One chief surgeon of a large hospital told me "Even if you prove it [that there is a relationship] in ten years, I won't believe it!" There seemed no particular reply I could make to that statement.*

Soon, however, I developed an excellent working relationship with Dr. Emanuel Revici and his Institute of Applied Biology, and for the next twelve years I worked full time with his patients.

---

*It was an honest statement at any rate. Twelve years later this surgeon announced that he had discovered a relationship between personality and cancer.

I started with psychological interviews (of two to eight hours in length) and various kinds of personality tests. As I progressed I reported my work in psychological and psychiatric journals. After a number of years, I moved very gradually into psychotherapy work with the patients of the Institute and of Trafalgar Hospital. It seemed to me then, and it still does, that the best way a professional can get to know people, their history and the world in which they live, is to be involved in a psychotherapy process with them. The stories of people with cancer that I present throughout this book are typical of the people I worked with for over thirty-five years.

The single thing that emerged most clearly during my work was the *context* in which the cancer developed. In a large majority of the people I saw (certainly not all), there had been, previous to the first noted signs of the cancer, a loss of hope in ever achieving a way of life that would give real and deep satisfaction, that would provide a solid *raison d'être*, the kind of meaning that makes us glad to get out of bed in the morning and glad to go to bed at night—the kind of life that makes us look forward zestfully to each day and to the future.

Often this lack of hope had been brought into being by the loss of the person's major way of relating and expressing himself or herself and the inability to find a meaningful substitute. Now the meaning of the statistics showing the higher likelihood of cancer in widows and widowers, regardless of age, began to be clear. Among the widowed were many who had made the spouse, the marriage, the central focus of their lives; it was what gave meaning to their existence, and after the spouse died they could find no other way to express themselves. Similar was the explanation for the fact that for men, the highest peak of cancer came shortly after retirement age, whether that age was sixty, sixty-five, seventy, or any other.* In married couples, the cancer mortality rate for both men and women was higher among those who had had no children than it was among those who did. I

*It was even true for those former Nazis who, in 1946 and 1947, were forcibly retired from the German bureaucratic service at thirty-five to forty years of age!

am certain the explanation of this is that when the relationship between the spouses was lost, but they stayed together for religious or other reasons, the children provided a good way of relating for many. It was also lower among those married couples who made the spouse the beneficiary of their insurance policies than those who did not!

I was able to make over thirty predictions on statistically reliable differences in cancer mortality rates in various groups. I could predict which groups would have a higher rate of loss of a major way of relating; according to my predictions, this group would also have a higher mortality rate. Whenever these predictions could be checked against published statistics, they were proved correct. (The professional publications on these findings are given in the Resource Directory.)

With many other individuals I saw and worked with, there had been no objective loss of a relationship, but there had been a loss of hope that the way that they used to express themselves, and the relationships they had, would ever give the deep satisfaction they wanted so much. No matter how successful they were, no matter how high they climbed in their profession, they found that it did not provide fulfillment. They could not find lasting zest and pleasure in their success and eventually had given up hope of *ever* finding it. The profound hopelessness was, in many of the people I saw, followed by the appearance of cancer. Over and over again I found that the person I was working with reminded me of the poet W. H. Auden's definition of cancer. He called it "a foiled creative fire."

As this pattern became clearer, I also began to work with *control groups,* people without cancer to whom I gave the same personality tests and worked with in the same way in psychotherapy. Over a period of many years, I found this pattern of loss of hope in between 70 and 80 percent of my cancer patients and in only 10 percent or so of the control group.

Sydney was a successful businessman whose high drive and a wide-ranging and quick intelligence had helped him achieve a very high position in his field. He had always believed in keeping the channels of promotion open in his company for new blood and new ideas, so, at sixty-five when he had been chief executive officer and chairman of the board for five years, he retired. When I asked him several years later what he had expected to do with his still-high energy level, he looked a little blank and said that he had thought tennis and golf would be wonderful and that now he would have had a chance to play as much as he wanted to.

Indeed for a year he did play both of these a good deal. He was a natural athlete and before World War II had played Class A baseball with a good chance of going to the major leagues; the draft and a stint in the paratroops ended this option. Sydney still played well and was much in demand from the members of a number of country clubs to play golf and tennis with them. Although he had looked forward to this life, it still left him unsatisfied and feeling increasingly empty and "drifting." He couldn't understand it; all his life he had loved sports and looked forward to the time when he would have enough leisure to spend all his time at them. Now it was somehow not enough. He was hungry for something, but did not know that.

Then Sydney went to Scotland with a group to play at one of the great golf courses there. At a luxurious hotel he played golf with a very congenial group every morning and tennis most afternoons. The weather was pure gold and wonderful. After five days he woke up one morning and found, to his shock and surprise, that he was wishing it would rain so that he would not have to continue his schedule.

At around this time he began to develop some digestive symptoms and after a medical workup was diagnosed as having cancer of the small intestine.

After finishing with both surgery and the course of chemotherapy that followed it, Sydney sat around the house a good deal, watching television and reading newspapers. He felt vaguely depressed and lost. Nothing interested him very much.

He felt tired and run-down all the time. A year after the chemotherapy was completed a new metastasis was found and a second
course was instituted.

During this period we began to work together. A friend of
Sydney's had suggested a consultation with me and he agreed.
We liked each other and began to work in ninety-minute sessions three or four times a month. That seemed to both of us
the most useful and meaningful pace for him.

Sydney's main problem was his constant tiredness. Rest did
not seem to help him. We discussed the fact that there are two
separate kinds of exhaustion. For acute exhaustion one needs
rest and sleep. For chronic exhaustion—such as he was suffering
from—an entirely different prescription is needed. What is required here is a change in the person's complete ecology—a
change in energy intake and outflow. Chronic exhaustion is
much more likely to be mostly caused by a blocked energy flow
than it is by a lack of energy. The tiredness is generally a result
of a lack of *available* energy due to blocked expression channels
rather than a result of a lack of energy in the organism. At one
point in our talks Sydney said to me: "It's true that taking it easy
does not restore my energy, even after months of it. I just get
more tired. I guess one trouble with doing nothing is that you
can't stop and rest!"

As we worked on and explored this area, it became increasingly plain that he had lost the context and meaning of his life.
Starting out in the heart of the Depression, and coming from
a poor family, he had focused his whole being on business. He
had loved it and brought to it a high drive and a high ethical
standard. It had been the center of his existence and gave him
purpose, a sense of himself, and a reason to get up in the
morning. Without this, nothing had any real meaning for him.
He felt that he could have borne any other loss and still, after
a time at any rate, gone on with his usual zest and enthusiasm.
I gave him the great speech of Shakespeare's Othello to read.
Othello has just come to the conclusion that the most meaningful thing in *his* life, his relationship with Desdemona, was lost
and that she had been unfaithful to him. He says that if he had

been wounded, unjustly accused of crimes, imprisoned, lost his position as general, or any other thing:

> Yet I could bear that too; well, well:
> But there, where I have garner'd up my heart,
> Where either I must live, or bear no life;
> The fountain from the which my current runs,
> Or else dries up; To be disgarded thence!

Sydney read it over once, line by line, getting the meaning. Then he read it again with deep feeling. "When you lose what is *real* for you," he said, "nothing else matters very much. You might as well be dead."

I pointed out that that was clearly how he felt and the message he was giving his body. I asked him how he could expect his immune system to mobilize itself and fight for his life under these circumstances. He agreed and asked, "Well, what can I do?" I replied that it was clearly time that he and I got to work.

Nothing seemed to have much meaning for Sydney. He felt that everything was somehow vague and meaningless; nothing had sharp emotional impact. He remembered how he had felt in earlier periods of his life, how he had been excited and involved. He could recall and even sometimes reinvoke these feelings, but they did not seem to apply to him now. The memories were there, but they were just memories. I quoted Edwin Arlington Robinson to him.

> I cannot find my way; there is no star
> In all the shrouded heavens anywhere;
> And there is not a whisper in the air
> Of any living voice, but one so far
> That I can hear it only as a bar
> Of lost imperial music. . . .

"Yes," he said, "yes. He knew."

We talked about the fact that there was nothing that really interested him, nothing that he wanted to do. He was just drifting and being passive about his life. I told him about a saying of Gurdjieff, one of the great esoteric teachers: "Energy expressed in a passive way is lost forever. Energy spent in active work is shortly transmuted into a fresh supply." It was no wonder, I said, that he was constantly so tired.

The basic answer we arrived at was that all his life Sydney had been interested in two things: physical expression in sports and business. Both of these were now closed down pretty much, and he could not really conceive of any other activities that could really engage him. Active sports participation was being made ever more difficult by the inexorable processes of aging and these were speeded up by his illness. As for business, it no longer held his interest. He had worked at it for many years, had encountered and dealt with most of the major problems involved, and had little real interest left in it.

We began to explore what was blocking Sydney's perception of other areas to which he could devote his energies. With an excellent intelligence and many abilities, that he could not find a way of expressing his creativity in such a rich and complex culture as ours surely indicated some pretty strong emotional blocks. As we explored and worked these through, went back to their sources and examined them together with adult eyes, Sydney's energy level began to rise. He had always been interested in foreign affairs and politics but had never become involved with either. Soon he began to read actively and widely, to take seminars offered to high-level businessmen and professionals, and to find others who were similarly interested and involved. Although he thought at first that he would get into politics, perhaps helping in the campaign of someone he thought would be good for the country, this did not materialize. Sydney began to realize that his interests were on other levels than those at which he had been looking—deeper and more philosophical. Presently he joined an organization similar to The Club of Rome, a group of very serious and intelligent people who were concerned with the long-term effects in our society of the population explosion, of the increasing average size of businesses and agricultural units, and issues of this sort.

It was a hardworking group that called for everything he had in experience and intelligence and more. Sydney was stretched to his limits and beyond. He began to study sociological issues and concepts. His energy level became almost as high as it had been when he was working his way up in business forty years before. Studying, discussing, arranging, and participating in seminars with social scientists on specific issues filled his life. I had to encourage him to keep up some golf and a regular exercise program in order to stay in shape. The second round of chemotherapy was successful and there have been no recurrences of his cancer in the past five years. Our sessions gradually stopped as they became harder and harder to schedule because of his involvement in his work. Now he is a fulfilled man; a man who is much too busy, much too *present* in his own life, to ask himself whether or not he is happy.

When I started psychotherapy work with people with cancer, I used the methods and concepts with which I had been trained. My background and orientation were very Freudian and psychoanalytic. (I belonged to that group which, if we did not bow toward Vienna every morning, it was probably because we were not sure in which direction it lay!) I had been trained in and used a modified psychoanalytic technique—we did not meet five times a week, and we sat in chairs instead of using a couch. Also I talked a good deal more than the classical psychoanalytic approach approved. However, my method was based on the Freudian concepts, and I saw things and interpreted the patients' comments in the way indicated by Freudian theory.

The people with cancer I was working with were cooperative and easy to get along with. They made no objections to my method and seemed to enjoy working with me. Gradually, however, I became aware that there were some major problems with my approach.

First, what we were talking about had very little to do with patients' present concerns. Here were people under the hammer of fate, often in physical pain, very often with deep anxieties and worries about the present and the future. They were concerned with their own mortality, with what would happen to their loved ones if they died, with how to decide between different treatment programs when it was a life-and-death decision and they had insufficient information and conflicting opinions from the experts, and with problems of this kind. As the theoretical model I was using subtly directed the process, very soon we were talking about early childhood experiences, toilet training, and the like. More and more it became plain to me that we were missing patients' real life experiences to talk about what theory indicated was important. What we were doing, it became increasingly plain, was irrelevant, and this at a time when the person with cancer had little time and energy to spare for irrelevancies.

A second problem with the approach was that I was constantly seeing things in my patients that had no place in the theoretical model I was using—that should not have existed, but did. In the psychoanalytic model there is no place for basic positive motives. Motives that are positive are seen as distortions of negative and unacceptable drives. Although this is how I had been trained to look at human beings, what I was seeing was quite different. I was seeing courage that was *not* a reaction formation to dependency and narcissism. I was seeing love for a spouse that was *not* oedipal displacement. I was seeing dignity that was bone-deep and not a reflection of something else. As I worked, I found myself respecting my patients more and more and I was increasingly proud to be a human being. These are not the emotions a Freudian-trained and -oriented therapist is supposed to have. I became increasingly convinced that something was very wrong with the model of a human being and with the therapy method I was using.

The third thing that made me understand that my therapeutic approach was not valid for these people was that none of my patients was getting better! They might look forward to my visits, they might even feel better afterward, but they kept right on dying at the same rate as if I were not involved with them at all. Psychotherapy was making no difference to their survival rate.

As I look back, I ought to have expected this. Every experienced therapist, working with one of the classical methods of dynamic psychotherapy, has had patients develop cancer at the end of or during an excellent therapeutic process. To make a difference, the therapy could not be one based on the models that were generally in use today.

I began to examine the basic premises of my approach and the psychological situation of the people with cancer with whom I was working. By the time Sydney and I started working together, a radically new approach had evolved: an approach that was relevant and felt relevant to the patients, was relevant to the context in which they had fallen ill, an approach that often stimulated the patients' immune system so that their response to the medical program improved.

Ever since I learned how to use this approach some twenty years ago, approximately half of my "hopeless," "terminal," patients have gone into long-term remission and are still alive. The lives of many others seemed longer than standard medical predictions would see as likely. Nearly all found that working in this new way improved the "color" and the emotional tone of their lives and made the last period of their lives far more exciting and interesting than they had been before starting the therapeutic process. This book is about this method, how it can be used by psychotherapists, how patients who are not working with a therapist can use the insights gained from the research to try to extend and improve their own lives, and how families and friends can help. I shall describe the approach briefly here. The rest of this book and the extensive individual stories of people I worked with are to illustrate it, and to make it useful for cancer patients, therapists, families, and friends.

Every psychotherapy process, early in its development, defines the basic questions it is trying to answer. In the usual models of therapy, there are three of these.

1. What is wrong with this person?

2. How did he or she get that way?

3. What can be done about it?

These questions are central to the therapy process, whether the therapist has been trained in a Freudian, a Jungian, an Adlerian, an Existentialist, or a Humanistic manner and model. Therapy based on these questions can be wonderful and effective for help with a wide variety of emotional or cognitive problems. It is, however, not effective with cancer patients. *It simply does not mobilize the person's self-healing abilities and bring them to the aid of the medical program.* We have now had enough experience in many different countries to state this as a fact.

The therapeutic approach developed in this research for work with people with cancer is based on entirely different questions. These are:

1. What is right with this person? What are his (or her) special and unique ways of being, relating, creating, that are his own and natural ways to live? What is his special music to beat out in life, his unique song to sing so that when he is singing it he is glad to get up in the morning and glad to go to bed at night? What style of life would give him zest, enthusiasm, involvement?

2. How can we work together to find these ways of being, relating, and creating? What has blocked their perception and/or expression in the past? How can we work together so that the person moves more and more in this direction until he is living such a full and zestful life that he has no more time or energy for psychotherapy?

As is immediately obvious, a psychotherapy based on this approach is quite different from one based on the older questions. Apart from anything else, it is more of an exciting adventure and has a different basic quality. We are looking for what is right with the patient, not what is wrong. I shall spend the rest of this book illustrating how the new method works.

When I began work, I simply added psychotherapy to the medical treatment. This, after I had learned how to work with people with cancer, often proved surprisingly effective. Over a period of time, however, my patients taught me that a wider approach was frequently a better one. Often they had been searching for a long time for ways to deal with their cancer and learned to work on all three levels of human life: the physical, the psychological, and the spiritual. I began to realize that those patients who had gone beyond me, who were consciously working on all three levels, tended to do better than those who were not. Over a period of time I learned about the holistic approach to illness and how to use it. In Chapter 6 I present my view of the matter as I see it now.

This is not completely a do-it-yourself book. For many people the approach outlined here goes much better when they are helped by a psychotherapist with the same orientation. I have also, however, included in this book a number of narratives about people who have done it themselves, with the help of family members or friends or an occasional counseling session.

One question that is frequently raised when I talk about psychological factors in the origin and development of cancer is "Does that mean that having cancer is a person's own fault?" My own strong and unequivocal response to this is "Certainly not!" All of us, as we develop in life, find ourselves entangled in emotional and intellectual traps. In our childhood we have so much to learn. Very early, with very limited experience and an unfinished brain, we have to learn such things as how to regard ourselves and others, what being a "good" person means, and how we can express our love and other feelings and seek love from others. Many other problems of this sort must also be solved in the first few years of life. Often we come to conclusions about the meaning of our parents' behavior that are dictated more by our being so young than they are by what our parents are or are not trying to communicate to us. So often we receive messages that were never sent and distort completely the meaning of our observations. Once we have come to a conclusion about how to solve such problems, these solutions tend to appear to us to be eternally true. They are certainly very hard to amend or correct.

Sometimes the traps we fall into on how to relate to ourselves and others are of such a nature that they put, over a long period of time, intolerable stress on our body. Sometimes partly as a result of this, the body breaks down. The cancer-defense mechanism may be weakened by these stresses.

According to the best theory we now have, we all get cancer many times each day. As the billions of our individual cells divide and multiply, some lose their coherence with the rest of the body—their ability to maintain their relation with the organ they are in is destroyed. We then have a cancer. This happens repeatedly, but the cancer-defense mechanism—we do not know very much about it specifically but we do know it exists—quickly takes care of the situation.

The strength of this defense mechanism, which is a part of

the immune system, is originally set by our genetic inheritance. While we are born with a defense mechanism of a certain strength, this strength can be weakened by a number of factors. Some types of coal-tar products can weaken it. Radiation can make it less effective. At least one type of long-term emotional stress can also lower its strength. The only type of emotional stress that we know of today that does this is the loss of hope that you can ever live your own life in a meaningful zestful way, that you can sing your own song in life and relate, be, create in the way most meaningful for you.

Part of my research was devoted to searching for an answer to the question of whether one can strengthen the cancer-defense mechanism, raise the effectiveness of the immune system, *after* a cancer has appeared. If we recover our hope for the ability to live our own life, will our cancer-defense mechanism recover its strength and come to the aid of the medical program? As we move toward living this life, will our own self-healing powers act more strongly and raise our "host resistance" to the cancer? The answer given by this research is a clear yes.

There are, of course, no guarantees here or anywhere else in life. Many of the patients discussed in this book died. Many, who had cancers that had not been responding to medical treatment, went into long remissions and are still alive. We do not know all the factors that made up the decision for each one about whether or not the cancer-defense mechanism could become strong enough so that the person could recover. Some of these factors are almost certainly physiological. Yet we do know enough of them now so that people with cancer have a new, an often effective way to fight for their lives.

2

AN INTRODUCTION TO THE METHOD: PSYCHOLOGICAL CHANGE TO MOBILIZE THE COMPROMISED IMMUNE SYSTEM

By every objective account Carol was indeed a successful woman. She had attained the highest rank that any woman ever had in her business field, becoming the first woman executive vice president of a large firm. She lunched with glamorous people at the most talked-about restaurants and lived in a penthouse on Fifth Avenue. Her family was very proud of her and her college classmates and friends regarded her with envy. The only thing wrong was that secretly she hated her life and everything about it. Particularly she disliked the people she worked with. When Carol was in her late thirties, her doctor, during a regular yearly physical examination, was disturbed to see six large black moles on her back that had not been there the previous year. He took a biopsy of one of them. When Carol returned three days later, he told her that they were malignant. Her prognosis, by any reasonable medical standards, was very poor.

She knew of my work through her secretary, whose sister had at one time consulted me. She left the physician's office, went to the nearest telephone, looked up my number, and called me. As I had free time, I saw her later that afternoon. We talked for an hour, liked each other, and set up a regular series of appointments.

In the fifth session, we had a discussion that I will never forget:

CAROL: Do you really believe in all this stuff that you have been handing me about everyone being different and needing to have their own individual life and to grow in their own way?

I: Yes, I really believe it.

CAROL: Then why haven't you listened to a word I've said?

I (*after a pause to think about it*): Obviously I've missed something very important that you have been saying. If you spell it out for me, I'll try my best to understand.

CAROL: Let's go back a moment first. How long are the sessions you have with patients?

I: An hour.

CAROL: What is the research on that? How do you know that that is the best amount of time for a session?

I: I don't know.*

CAROL: Okay, leave that. How many times a week do you see someone like me?

I: As a rule, twice a week. Sometimes once, and rarely, in special times and situations, perhaps three times.

CAROL: That's a pretty Procrustean bed, isn't it? Everyone, no matter how different they are or what their special ways of learning or growing, has to fit into your definition of the correct length of a session and the correct number of sessions a week.

---

*Later I checked and, of course, there is no such research. Apparently the time was first chosen because it was the easiest time for the therapist to schedule appointments—on the hour or half hour. More recently, when therapists decided that they would like a ten-minute break between appointments, they went to fifty minutes, again with no research. Then, in order to schedule more patients and increase their incomes, to forty-five minutes. The end of this sequence remains to be seen.

I: I guess I've never thought about it in these terms before. I'm learning something.

CAROL: I've told you at least three times how *I* learn. It has nothing to do with your schedule. Are you really interested in *my* schedules, or was that all talk?

I: Tell me again.

CAROL: I learn things in crash programs. I always have. If you want to do it my way, here's how it would go. We'll meet five or six times a week for a while. Then, and I'll tell you when, I'll take a vacation and go home and digest what we've covered. And don't call me, I'll call you. When I'm ready, I'll come back for another crash program. Now, do you mean all that shit you've been giving me about respecting and nurturing differences or do we do it in your regular way?

I *(after muttering weakly something about being hoist by one's own petard)*: We'll do it your way.

As is plain from this, Carol was a pleasure to work with. Clear, strong, and open, she tackled the exploration with vigor, humor, and strength.

Among the first things we covered was her contempt for herself for not being married. In the subculture she grew up in, a woman was supposed to get married by twenty-one or twenty-two or else consider herself an old maid and a failure as a human being. Carol had never gotten over this. We explored her feelings and how the message had been given to her that this was the only right way for a woman to live her life. Then one day we both began to giggle over what we had found out. She *didn't want* to get married. She enjoyed having affairs, preferably long-term ones, but she liked the man to go home after a sexual interlude. She liked to wake up in the morning alone "and have my coffee and read the paper in peace without some big galump messing up the place and wanting eggs and bacon and wanting to *talk* in the morning!" After the healing winds of laughter had blown through her feelings in this area, the tension and self-contempt gradually disappeared.

We talked at length about her job. She *hated* it. She heartily disliked the people who rose to the top in her field and worried that working with them would make her as unfeeling, driven, and ruthlessly ambitious as they were. She despised the fang-and-claw nature of the corporate world. Her very high level of ability had taken her far. It had been recognized and had protected her in the organization intrigues from which she had rigorously abstained. (And, Carol said, she was also helped by the fact that the organization felt it helped their image to have a "token woman" in a high position.) But she dreaded becoming a part of the system. Further, she had found out that her ability and her willingness to work to the limit had brought her neither happiness nor inner peace. She felt at a dead end; she had done the best she could and the result showed only a future of more work to her limit and no feelings of being worthwhile. I quoted to her the opening line from *The Divine Comedy*, "In the middle of the journey of our life, I found myself in a dark wood, where the straight path was lost." She smiled sadly and nodded in agreement. This was she.

I kept concentrating not only on what Carol did *not* like, but also on what she did. What were the best moments of her life? Was there any work she had enjoyed, felt at home in? What work had used her in the right way? When had she most often felt the "good tired," not the "yuck tired"? When and where had she had those periods in which you suddenly look up, three hours have gone by, you missed lunch and never noticed? You feel tired, but good, "put together and whole," relaxed and somewhat charged up at the same time? I kept her coming back to these questions.

The college she had gone to had had extended outside study periods during which students work regularly in a job for a semester. The students live off campus during this time. During one such period Carol had worked at a center for retraining physically handicapped adults. These adults, who had been severely hurt in accidents or through illness, were being physically rehabilitated as far as possible, retaught living skills, and taught new vocational abilities. Carol had been deeply involved with her work there and had loved it. College, when she returned to it, had seemed rather "pale."

She felt that doing this kind of work would be something she would enjoy and that would really fulfill her. However, to change from her present life-style and work to become a Special Education teacher seemed so overwhelming as to be impossible. How could one even begin to explore it?

We began with the "What is the first thing to do?" game. The first thing to do seemed to her to get some education in the field. The first thing to do was to take some evening courses to find out how she really would feel about this kind of work now—at her present stage of development. The first thing to do was to find out what colleges near her had such courses. And so on. It turned out that the first thing to do in changing her life was to buy three stamps on the way home to write some nearby colleges for catalogs!

Carol took several evening courses over the next year and found that this field did still deeply interest and engage her. Then, to the absolute horror and dismay of her parents and to the astonishment and disapproval of her siblings and her friends, she resigned from her job, sold her penthouse, moved into a walk-up near the college she had chosen, and became a full-time graduate student.

Carol enjoyed the courses very much and the internship even more. She found that she enjoyed getting up in the morning and going to school or work and that her life had a far more enjoyable "color" than it had for the years she had been in business. Gradually the periods between our "crash courses" grew longer and longer. One day she told me: "I'm beginning to phase you out. Bill [a friend from the college with whom she was having an affair—one in which he would leave her apartment at two or three in the morning and go back to his own!] is better than you are to talk about my work, and Nora [also a friend from the college] is better than you are to talk about Bill!"

We tapered off the work, and after some time I lost sight of her. Ten years later I met her bounding jauntily along the street. It was "big hug" time as we greeted each other and talked for a moment. We were both in a hurry for appointments, however, and soon Carol continued on her way. After a few steps, however, she turned back and called me. She asked, "Do you know why I've never gotten in touch with you?" I shook my head, no. She went on: "It's because I've been too busy living my life to have any time for any such nonsense as cancer, psychotherapy, or you!" For a psychotherapist that was a combination of the Congressional Medal of Honor and the Nobel Prize. There could not have been a finer reason.

A few last notes to this story should be added. For the first few months we worked together, the black melanoma moles on her back seemed to be increasing in size slowly. As there was nothing to do about that, we did nothing. The growth seemed to stop (according to her oncologist who inspected them regularly) after a few months. About six months later they seemed to be shrinking. This continued until they were no longer visible to the eye. They did not reappear for the next fifteen years. To my knowledge, and I believe she would call me if there was more trouble of this kind, she is still cancer-free over twenty years later.

I met her again about seven years after the encounter described above. We were both at a Lincoln Center concert. We talked over coffee afterward. She had stayed in Special Education for about fifteen years and then felt it was time for a change. She was growing and changing and felt that it was time for a new adventure. She decided that she would enjoy using some of her administrative and managerial skills, but in a new and different way. She was now executive director of a large charitable foundation. She said that she enjoys this very much and looks forward to going to work each day. She felt that her life was full, rich, and meaningful.

From the viewpoint of the usual approach to psychotherapy today, this case history is quite unusual. There was much stress on Carol's health and very little stress on her pathology. When neurotic aspects of her personality were explored, the exploration was kept in the context of their being factors blocking her perception and expression of her best and most enjoyable ways of creating, being, relating. The psychotherapeutic process was clearly oriented toward searching together for her zest and enthusiasm, not for the causes of her problems. Once this orientation was made clear to Carol, she and I kept each other on the track and reinforced each other.

This was not the kind of psychotherapy I had been originally trained to do and certainly not what I had expected to do at the start of this research. I was forced to move toward this approach if I wished to help my patients with cancer mobilize their self-healing mechanisms and bring them to the aid of the medical treatment. Psychotherapy based on the usual approach simply did not do this; therapy based on this approach was far more likely to accomplish this aim. Further, where it did not succeed in helping the patient respond successfully to the medical protocol, it—in the great majority of cases—did succeed in changing the *color* and flavor of the person's last period of life in a positive direction.

The rest of this chapter is a discussion of the method illustrated by the story of Carol and how it can be used by others. I have concentrated, here on how it is used in a psychotherapy process, but the ideas and concepts are also valid for those consciously working on their own growth and becoming in other ways.

Years ago we used to do a particular kind of experiment in the psychology laboratories. We would tell our subjects that we were doing research in free association and ask them to respond freely to a list of words we presented one by one. Unknown to the subject, the therapist would have a "preferred category" of responses in mind. These might be something like "nature objects," "plurals" (responses that included more than one object or process—"glasses" rather than "glass"), responses indicating movement, or whatever. Whenever the subject's response fell into the favored category for this particular session, the experimenter would also respond. In one study he would say approvingly "mm-hmm," in another he would just tap his pencil before he recorded the response, in another he would incline his head slightly forward and back, and so forth. Only very rarely would subjects become conscious of the fact that this was not a bona fide study in free association. Almost invariably, however, they started responding more and more in the favored category until, after a comparatively short time, their responses were almost entirely within the favored category and they themselves were unaware of this. As we compare these studies to the therapeutic situation, an obvious difference is that by and large psychotherapists have far more prestige in patients' minds than experimenters in the psychology laboratories have in subjects' minds. Indeed, so great is psychotherapists' prestige and influence that individuals who have had a Freudian analysis continue to have Freudian dreams years after their analysis has been completed, those who have had a Jungian analysis, Jungian dreams, and so on with Adlerian, Existentialist, and almost certainly all other therapy systems.

Every experienced psychotherapist is aware that the goal of a nondirective or nondirected therapy is completely unobtainable. What therapists respond to in the patient's behavior and how the response is made, what is *not* responded to, and the therapists' behavior and even office arrangement, all give strong if subtle cues to the assumptions on which the process is based and its orientations and goals. By their behavior, both verbal and nonverbal, therapists clearly communicate to patients what the therapy is trying to accomplish and how the process is designed to bring about those effects. It is not possible, we know today, for therapists to mask their assumptions and goals. They must engage in some behavior, and this behavior is also communication.

———— ▬▬▬ ————

In any psychotherapy program, a central question, or set of questions, is being asked. These questions may or may not have been clearly verbalized by the participants, but they nevertheless guide and direct the course of the process. Whatever the different orientations and expectations of the patient and therapist before they begin, they soon come to an agreement about what these questions are even if they have never spoken directly of them. The interaction between the participants in the therapy process smooths out the differences in what they are searching for, and by a series of verbal and nonverbal cues they begin to dance to the same kind of music and move toward the same goals.

The basic questions of classical psychodynamic psychotherapy were set by Freud. Others had speculated about these as the basis of a possible approach to psychological pathology, but when Freud built the foundations of modern psychotherapy he set them into its very bone structure.

Freud was a neurologist before he was a psychiatrist. The basic questions of neurology are: *"What are the symptoms? What is the hidden lesion that is causing them? What can we do about the lesion, or failing that, how can we teach the person to compensate for it?"* Freud took these as the basic questions of the new psychological therapy he was inventing. In it, he asked, *"What are the symptoms? What is the hidden lesion that is causing them? What can we do about it, either to remove the lesion or to help the person compensate for it?"* Instead of physical lesions, Freud now looked for psychological lesions.

There is no question of the tremendous usefulness of this formulation for the development of psychotherapy, or of the fact that it has given us a method to treat many painful and disabling syndromes whose primary symptoms were psychological or physical or both. Nearly everything we know of psychotherapy today rests on these formulations of Freud.

However, long experience, both of mine and of many others working in this field, has shown that *this is not a useful basic set of questions when we are working with people who have cancer. It simply does not lead to patients' mobilizing their own healing resources and bringing them to the aid of the medical program.* If this is one of the goals of the psychotherapist, then he or she must find another set of basic questions. At this point in our search for knowledge, this is not speculation, but understanding based on long, hard experience.

These days, when the ideas of psychotherapy are so well known, almost invariably patients clearly expect that the purpose of psychotherapy is to find out what is wrong with them, how they got that way, and what can be done about it. They come in well prepared to search with the therapist for the explanation of their symptoms (in their past, their present, and how they are reacting to it, or—among the more sophisticated patients—in a combination of their past and their present). Media presentations of psychotherapy, widely read literature on the subject, and the talk of friends who have been through the process have generally provided these usually accurate expectations and demands. The therapist, with the same cultural background, which was heavily reinforced by professional training, also almost invariably has the same expectations.

Therapist and patient today may differ in sophistication but are usually pretty close to each other in their viewpoint of the basic structure and basic question of the process. Patients are a little more likely than professionals still to be under the influence of the concept (so well portrayed in the movie *Spellbound*) that the hidden lesion consists of one traumatic incident and that when this is uncovered and the resulting emotions purged they will be freed of their symptoms. Therapists are a bit more likely to see the traumatic incident as an example of how the patient saw the relationship between the world and himself, and how this led to the present psychological situation, but the basic agreement about the neurologically based questions is still there.

With this mutual, usually unverbalized, viewpoint and therefore with much mutual reinforcement about what the therapy is searching for and attempting to do, the process tends to move inexorably in the direction Freud organized. We, in our post-Freudian age, tend to accept this as the natural way therapy works. It is indeed the conventional wisdom on the subject and has been strengthened by innumerable novels, short stories, television presentations, and personal accounts.

Under these conditions, it is very hard for therapists to change their approach. Not only must they reexamine their training and reevaluate their experience, they are also going counter to the beliefs of their culture and to the expectations of their patients. Nevertheless, if therapists want to enable their cancer patient clients to bring the best of their self-healing and self-repair abilities to the aid of the medical treatment (in the currently accepted terms, "to help mobilize their immune systems"), this is precisely what they have to do.

We have learned that there is another set of questions that can serve as the basis of the psychotherapeutic process and that *does* help clients increase their host resistance to the cancer. These new questions are far removed from the neurological approach, which tends to be little interested in those areas of patients that are functioning well and cause no symptoms. They are the questions of what is *right* with clients, what is their most natural way of being, relating, creating. What kind of life and life-style would make them glad to get up in the morning and glad to go to bed at night, would give them the maximum zest and enthusiasm in life? Would use all of them so that on physical, psychological, and spiritual levels they would express themselves in ways syntonic and "natural" to their entire being? What kind of life would they be living if they adjusted the world to themselves instead of—as our patients generally have done—adjusted themselves to the world?

"Let us suppose," we say in effect to a patient, "that your

Fairy Godmother will come in that door in a few minutes. She will make you an offer. In six months your inner and outer life can be exactly what you would like it to be so that you would use yourself most completely and have the maximum enjoyment and zest possible. You can change your feelings and your circumstances. There are no limitations on age, sex, education, and so forth. We shall assume that you choose good physical health as a basis and take it from there. There are only two catches. You must tell her in the next five minutes, and this is a once-in-a-lifetime deal. She won't be back after granting your proposal."

Therapy that is useful for mobilizing cancer patients' immune systems aims at discovering the answer to this question and understanding what has blocked its perception and/or its being lived out as a life-style. And then helping patients move toward it.

Very often patients will respond with "I don't know" when asked how they could change their life. The goal then becomes having them accept that this is the most important question at this stage of their life. Mere acceptance of the question and a commitment to finding out the answer frequently have a positive effect on patients' immune systems. I have seen patients who began to respond better and more effectively to their medical protocol when they made and emotionally accepted the commitment.

The therapist must have a clear understanding of the new questions and must communicate them repeatedly to the patient until they reinforce each other in their quest for finding out what is right with the client, not what is wrong with him or her.

One patient with a metastasized breast cancer put it, at the end of the seventh session: "What I hear you saying is that I have lived my life as if I bought my clothes off the rack. They fitted pretty well, but were standard issue. And that if I want to set my immune system an example I have to start living my life as if I were having my clothes made especially for me by a top-level couturier—clothes and a life that is designed specifically for me, not for someone approximately my size who wants to fit in with everyone else and be wearing whatever is fashionable at the moment. That if I really get committed to this, then it will be as if my immune system looks up, says, 'Oh, this specific individual is worth fighting for. Why didn't you say so before?' I've got to set my body an example by taking care of me and gardening who *I* am, not just adjusting myself to whatever is on the clothing rack of life."

After warning that there are no guarantees that the approach will succeed in reversing the cancer's course, but that the game is worth the candle in any case, I agreed with this metaphor.

What we are doing here is changing the basic definition of psychotherapy. In the past, it has been a process of removing a patient's special pain and disabilities, of reducing the symptoms. The definition we are using here is essentially that of the psychiatrist Karen Horney: "A process in which the uniqueness, the individuality, the neurosis itself, is moved from the front of a patient's face where it acts as blinders and moved to the back of the neck where it acts as an outboard motor!"

In this approach, the search for pathology and its roots are secondary. Primary is the search for what would be a zestful and enthusiastic life for *this* person.

Certainly pathology must often be explored and worked through. But *it is viewed in context* as the process that blocks the perception and the expression of the individual's special song to sing in life; as the cause of his or her loss of contact with enthusiasm and joy. This puts it in an entirely different view, and the therapeutic process has a different flavor and different results.

This type of therapy depends on a real "encounter," a real contact between therapist and client. The therapist must, moreover, *care* intensely, believe in the importance of and be involved in the special growth, the individual becoming, of the patient. By his or her faith, the therapist tries to lead the patient to give up fears and anxieties, concern about "success" and the opinions of others, and ultimately become concerned about his or her own authentic development.

There are certainly some individuals who can embark on this exploration without the aid of a psychotherapist. To use an old analogy, it is better, if you are crossing a mountain range, to have an experienced guide who knows the area and has been over it before. However, some people have crossed it alone, some in groups and some with maps (in the form of books like this, techniques such as specially adapted meditations, and so forth). However, many of us need a good guide.

"Come now," we might say to a patient, "let us suppose that God is an existentialist! One day an Angel comes to visit you. The Angel says that they have learned long ago that they must design an individual Heaven for each arrival there. There is no particular hurry in your case, but their computers are down and they are trying to stay as far ahead as they usually do. Therefore they are asking each person to design his or her own Heaven. How would you design a way of life for you that you will enjoy for a long period of time? One in which you will relate, create, give, take, express yourself, in the right way for you, the way that you are built and designed for?"

Obviously this particular phrasing would be used with people of particular intellectual backgrounds. However, the general approach is not so conditioned. I have, as the case histories scattered throughout this book indicate, used it with individuals of a very wide variety of economic, social, and educational backgrounds with equal success.

"Or suppose," we might say, "you suddenly find out that there is reincarnation and that furthermore you can choose now how and where you will be reincarnated. The choice is yours and you can direct your future life from here. Tell me about your choice. It is an entire life that you are setting yourself up for so make sure it is one that you would enjoy."

Or "Let's look at your life as a novel of which you were the author. Now the publisher calls you and says that they want to bring out a second edition. It is a curious and unusual fact of this particular publishing house that you have to live through whatever you write. They say it keeps their writers on their toes! Let's you and I get into the rewrite. First, what are the things you want to change for the second edition? Then we will talk about the things you want to keep the same."

Or perhaps something on the line of "Let's us, you and I, pretend for a while that you really care about yourself. That you are a friend to you and know you *very* well and love you. And that you—as this friend—have the power to give a gift of a year: to organize a year for you that would be the best gift you can design; that would give you the best year possible. Tell me about what the year would be like."

Or "As you look at life, what were the best moments? What were those moments that you remember as the peak ones?" After exploring these, the therapist goes on to help the patient find what the moments had in common and what themes of this particular individual's life history they celebrated and expanded. Then the exploration goes on to how a life could be set up, what it would be like, so that there would be as many of these moments as possible.

There is, in this approach, as much, and usually more, emphasis on the good moments in the patient's life as on the bad moments. What was enjoyed the most? What courses in high school or college were the best? A contrast is sought between the best and the worst moments so that both may be understood and their relationships to *this person's* personality seen. From this one continues to building an understanding of the kind of life that would fulfill this person the most.

Much of the success of this approach rests on the therapist's ability to keep in mind its goals and keep the process oriented toward them. It is vital that patients be brought in on this—that they too have a sense of the goals.

Over the last dozen years, I frequently have received a letter or phone call with the following thrust. "I have cancer and I have read your book *You Can Fight for Your Life.* I want to work with a therapist with this point of view, as I feel that it definitely applies to me. How do I find a therapist who will work with me from this viewpoint? I live in a small city in Missouri (or the far Dakotas, or in France, or New Zealand)."

I have generally answered along the following lines. "Find the experienced and seasoned therapists in your area. Ask the local medical society and the local psychological organization. Assuming that they are trained people, then start a shopping procedure. See them one at a time until you find one that you like. Someone with whom the 'chemistry' is good, and whom you would like to have as a friend. You may have to see a number of them. That is the first essential. Unless there is liking, you may get somewhere, but it will take you nine times as long and be nine times as hard.

"When you find one like that, give him a copy of the book. Ask if he can work with you from this viewpoint—from the viewpoint of finding out what is right with you, not what is wrong. Is the therapist willing to make a compact with you? Then when *you* lose the thread and start searching for what is wrong with you, he will remind you that you are off the track. And when *he* reverts to the older method, you remind him."

I generally finish by saying that I will be glad to discuss specific problems with both of them in a conference call if they wish. A number of people to whom I have written in this way have later told me that the therapy process was richly rewarding. There have been a few telephone calls and some occasional supervision on my part. Presently, I believe that there will be enough therapists who comprehend this method that such letters to me and the necessity for my supervision will no longer be required.

When people with cancer are presented with this concept and set of goals, their negative reactions frequently fall into one or more of three classes:

1. "If I found my own music, it would be so discordant that I wouldn't like it and no one else could stand it either. My own 'natural' way of being is ugly and repellent, and I learned a long time ago not to express it if I wanted to have *any* relationships or be able to live with myself."

2. "If I found my own song and tried to sing it, I would find there was no place in this world for anyone like me." (The major variation here is "I couldn't support myself if I was living the song that is right for me.") "And it would be so bitter to know it and not be able to sing it that I'd rather not know."

3. "My own song would have such contradictions built into it that it would be impossible." (As one patient put it, "I'd really like to be a hermit with a harem!")

Essentially patients are saying that if they find their own music, it would either be so ugly that it would not be acceptable to themselves or others, or not possible to play in this society, or else impossible because of its self-contradictory nature.

In more than twenty-five years of using this approach, I have seen these reactions many, many times. Yet I have *never* seen a single person who, upon finding his or her own song and style, still felt the same. With all the people with whom I have worked, their own song was one that was acceptable to them and others, was possible to play fully in this culture (and to make a living at when this was necessary), and increased their human relationships and made them more fulfilling. In addition, in every case the song was socially positive and acceptable. *I have never seen an exception to this.* The following case histories will serve as examples of what I am saying. (Of course, everyone who voices the objections tends to believe that they apply only in their own case.)

No matter what the special music of *this* person appeared to be at first look, on deeper examination it was positive, possible, and socially acceptable. One example was Pedro.

I first met Pedro while I was making rounds in the hospital in 1960. He was a Hispanic, slim and attractive, looking about nineteen or twenty. Each day he greeted us courteously and responded to questions quietly while managing to make it perfectly clear that he had absolutely no respect for, nor expectations from, us middle-class, middle-age whites. I was fascinated by the manner in which he indicated his attitude. This man had style! I resolved to see if I could breach the obvious barrier and work with him. One day on rounds, I asked him if I could come to see him late that afternoon and talk with him for a while. He replied with perfect courtesy, "It's your hospital. I'm sure you can do as you please." At four that day I went in to see him.

Pedro and I talked several times a week for a number of months and got to know and to like each other. Gradually I began to have a sense of what his life had been.

He had been raised in the South Bronx, an area containing a mixture of blacks and Hispanics. His mother had had three children; her husband, the father of the first, had deserted her; the father or fathers of the next two were not known to Pedro. The mother, warm and loving, had been so busy and worked such long hours trying to support, house, and feed the children that she had had no time to supervise them.

At nine, Pedro joined one of the youth gangs in the neighborhood. It was a necessary survival step for a young person growing up in that area. In the gang he came into his own. He felt as if that were where he belonged. As he put it, "They . . . were *right* for me." He rose rapidly through the ranks and by sixteen had reached the highest position in the gang hierarchy. This was the position of "warlord," or dictator, during those times when the gang was having periods of physical conflict with another gang.

Soon what happens to many gangs happened to his. Some of the brothers were arrested, some died on the streets, some were drafted into the army, some moved away, some married and left the gang. Pedro was left alone on the streets. For a time he hung around the same places and even engaged in some of the same illegal activities, but life had lost its savor. He was offered membership in one of the adult criminal groups that had its headquarters in the area, but he turned it down. "It felt like some sort of dead end. I didn't feel right with those people." Approximately a year after the gang had finally dissolved, he came down with a rapidly progressing Hodgkin's disease and after another six months wound up in the hospital in which I was working.

At that time, this was a fatal disease. The Hodgkin's Institute in New York City did not have a single case of five years' survival. Since then, of course, there has been a tremendous change. Because of advances in chemotherapy, a person with Hodgkin's disease now has an 85 percent chance of long-term remission.

Here was a person who had had an "ideal" (from the viewpoint of his personality) way of being, relating, creating. It was now closed off. My belief was—and is—that in this culture there is room for every individual to express his or her natural ways of being, and that these ways would also be (1) socially positive and (2) improve human relationships in the ways most suited to the individual. If ever anyone seemed to be testing the last parts of this theory, it was Pedro!

At one time I asked him if he could tell me what had been so attractive, so right about the gang life. He explained it to me. "There was this group of men, see, and they *cared* about each other. No matter how much you argued and fought with each other, you always knew you could depend on the brothers. They were there for you when you needed them and you were there when they needed you." Pedro went on to describe the rhythm of gang life. There were long quiet periods when the members just relaxed, loafed, smoked, boasted about their exploits, and occasionally got into long, lazy discussions and sometimes arguments about sports. Then there were periods of intense excitement and danger when each man depended on the others for safety and survival.

I kept wondering what sort of socially positive work had a similar life-style. As we talked about this, it became clear to both of us that what he was describing was like the life of a firefighter. As Pedro and I discussed it, he became very interested and excited about this type of career. It was the first time he had ever shown the slightest interest in any type of work. We began to plan. The first thing we found out when we sent for the requirements was that a high school diploma was necessary. Pedro had left school unofficially in the eighth grade and officially two years later. In the hospital, he sent for the necessary correspondence courses to work for his equivalency diploma. And he began to work hard at them.

About this time, Pedro began to respond positively to the experimental chemotherapy program he was on—a program he had not responded to previously that was being continued only because nothing else was available and this, at least, had no negative side effects. Two years later this treatment protocol was abandoned as not useful. Soon he left the hospital and continued on outpatient status. He and I kept up our regular meetings.

Next was the problem of a job history. He could hardly put down on his job application that he had been the warlord of a street gang and then had had Hodgkin's disease! I managed to obtain some work recommendations for him from friends of mine, and he got a job in the stockroom of a small company. He was well liked there and worked hard. After a few months, he took the head of his department into his confidence and managed to get from him a letter of recommendation stating he had worked there for several years. He and I put together a work history that accounted for the rest of his time.

By now the hospital radiologist was in on the plot. Pedro was still on medication and was getting a chest X ray every month. After one of these, the radiologist called us both in, hung up the X-ray film on the viewing screen, and said, "You see that tiny spot on the sternum? That's all that's left of the Hodgkin's disease and unless you knew exactly what you were looking for, you'd almost certainly never see it. They'll *never* spot this. Go take the physical." Pedro did, passed it, and six months later was appointed as a firefighter.

That was over twenty years ago. Pedro went off all medication over eighteen years ago. The cancer has never reappeared. Since that time he has married and has had several children. He loves his work and his life.

For a time, he used to drop into the office occasionally. Always unexpectedly (I never *could* convince him to make appointments!). I would shuffle my schedule whenever I could and we would talk and have some coffee or a beer together. Once in a while, if I was in the neighborhood, I would drop into the firehouse for a visit. Then we lost touch.

Fifteen years later Pedro came back to see me. He said he had a problem. He had been told that if he took the examination for Lieutenant, he would be certain to pass it and to be appointed. His wife, children, and colleagues wanted him to take it. It would, however, mean a completely different life-style. He would be much more removed from the group of men, be doing much more paperwork, and the like. He felt he did not want this. He didn't want to take chances with his way of life; his body that somatized conflicts too well for risks to be acceptable. Both of us understood that in the future he would almost certainly change and want to follow a path that was different from the one he chose right now. We looked and found a way that he could turn down the examination without prejudice and still be able to apply for the job in the future if he wanted to. We then talked about his life during the past fifteen years. He was happy in his work and at home and was obviously a competent and confident man. We parted with warm affection and I expect, someday, to hear he has been made a lieutenant.

Not only was Pedro's dream acceptable to him and richly rewarding, it was also possible, no matter how unlikely it looked at first, to be lived out in this society. Literally the person could have it *and* make a living at it. Harold is a good example of this.

Harold was sixty-two with a cancer of the lymphatic system. He had a high school education and had, all his life, been a salesman in clothing stores. He had never married but had had a number of long-term and moderately intense relationships with women. He enjoyed reading, particularly about travel and adventure stories. His vacations were generally spent on the beach, sunning and swimming and watching the ocean.

As we explored together, there seemed to be no question about his dream. He wanted to be a physician. This had been his dream even as a young man, but he had had to go to work early and had not been able to afford college, let alone medical school.

On the surface, this dream seemed impossible to realize. If ever a dream seemed to test my belief that there was a way for each person to live out his or her natural and "right" way of living within our society, this was it.

Today Harold is working full time and loves his work. His supervisors think very highly of him and sometimes try to persuade him that working nine to five is enough and that he does not really need to arrive at eight or stay to six.

As I was working with Harold, we began to investigate what being a physician meant to him. What was, as he saw it, a physician's life like? What was its basic structure? To Harold, being a physician meant that people would come to him with their problems. Sometimes they would not be sure what these problems were, they would just know that they needed something or that something was wrong.

He would have the resources and training to be able to help them and to define and solve their problems. I asked him about short- and long-term relationships. Did he want to work with the same people over a period of time or have a constant stream of new ones? He preferred the latter. In other words, if he had been a physician he would have been an emergency room specialist and not a family physician, an internist, or a pediatrician.

As you come off the big north–south highway that runs up and down the Atlantic coast, at one particular point, near one of the resort cities, there is a sign that reads TOURIST INFORMATION. THIS WAY. Harold now works in the information booth. Some time ago I visited him. As I sat in the back of the booth, a car drew up with a family inside and the driver got out, came into the booth, and said, "Can you tell me where we can get a motel for a week? Near the beach." Harold began to ask questions. What did they enjoy doing on vacation? Were the children old enough to play on the beach alone or did they need constant supervision? In a few minutes the rest of the family were all in the booth and, under Harold's skillful questioning, were defining together for the first time, exactly what they wanted. At the end of a half hour they had completely defined what would be the ideal place for them and Harold had made a phone call and reserved rooms for them. I have rarely seen a person so clearly doing the job he was designed for nor one so fulfilled by his work.

Very often people object that they cannot possibly change their lives in a positive direction. They correctly point out that they are very ill, or that they have deep commitments with others depending on them, or they say that society will not permit it. I have never worked with anyone where positive change and growth, change that would make a critical difference in the individual's life experience, was impossible.

———————

Nor did I ever work with anyone who did not have a unique song to sing, a completely individual music to beat out, which, when it was found, had these three characteristics: It was joyful for the person, socially positive, and improved his or her human relationships. Of all the patients I have seen, the one who tested this most severely was Minnie.

Minnie was born in Eastern Europe toward the end of the last century. At that time, in emigrating families it was a custom for the father to come over first, leaving his wife and children until he could establish himself in the United States and send for them. Minnie's father emigrated when she was nine. There were three younger children. A few months after the father left, the mother died suddenly.

With the help of the local community (the *stetl*), Minnie took care of the younger children and, when she was ten or eleven, left the country, following the illegal border guide across the marshes with the children each holding tight to a knotted cord tied to her waist. The father met them in the United States. Apparently he was a rather weak, inadequate man who never was able to make much of a living. The quality of Minnie's early life may be indicated by her memory of saying to her father, "Poppa, the children are hungry." And his reply, "Tell them to bite their tongues. What could be better than a tongue sandwich?"

Minnie had one year of school in this country and then went to work in a needle-trades factory. With little help from her father, she raised the younger children and saw them all through college. By this time the father had died and presently Minnie married—a weak, inadequate man who never could make much of a living. Minnie had three children and continued to work almost constantly in the garment factories. The husband died after about fifteen years of marriage, and Minnie worked hard enough to help all three children through college. All became professionals. For a time, Minnie followed the younger one around in his jobs and kept house for him, but she realized he wanted to be independent. Minnie moved into a single-room occupancy hotel in New York City and spent her time looking out the window, taking walks on Broadway, looking at the shops, and listening to the radio. After less than a year of this life, she developed a cancer of the stomach and wound up in the hospital where I was working. (This was a "court of last resort," a place where people came when mainline medicine had nothing more to offer and where they could try an early experimental form of chemotherapy.)

Everyone loved Minnie. She was always good-tempered and agreeable. Her bed and bedside table were always neat and clean. No patient was easier to get along with. When asked how she was doing, she always gave the proper answer of a "good" patient: "I'm feeling better today."

Getting to know her on rounds, I too came to love Minnie. We started to work together. It became clear to me that she was a high-energy woman who had been extremely active all her life. Now there was no place for all the energy to go. All her life she had taken care of people so that the first and obvious suggestion was that she continue this: there were plenty of needs in a city like New York for someone with her giving abilities. Hospitals needed someone to give tender loving care to children, social agencies had various similar needs, and so on. It was the first time (and the only time) that I ever saw Minnie get angry. She had had it up to her ears taking care of people.

I began to search further. What was the lost dream? Where and when had it been lost? What was Minnie's natural talent for being and creating; the talent that if she could find it now would be the way for her to use her energy and intelligence, and her abilities that had never been tapped? The more we looked together, the clearer it became that there was nothing there.

According to my theory, all people have a natural way of being, relating, creating; when they find it, they are using themselves in the way most fulfilling to themselves. And all my experience had been that when they become committed to finding and then to living this new way, the body's defenses increase their functioning, and they frequently begin to respond much more positively to whatever medical treatment they are on. With Minnie, not only could I find no trace of this other way of being and creating, but she was slowly and steadily going downhill physically.

For every scientist it is clear that when the theory collides with the brute fact, it is the theory that must give way. My theory had run into an exception and was going to have to be drastically modified if not abandoned completely. I continued to work with Minnie because you do not abandon a patient when your theory is proved wrong. I knew she had come to look forward to and enjoy our sessions.

One day the Danish Royal Ballet came to town. It was a complete sellout. However, a friend had gotten me a ticket to an afternoon performance at the last minute. I called Minnie and asked if we could put off our three o'clock appointment until the next morning. She was as agreeable as ever and went on at some length that any time was fine with her and that it was so wonderful of me to see her so often, and so on.

The next morning when I saw her, I told her the reason for the cancellation. And then I discovered Minnie's secret!

When she was thirteen and then again when she was fifteen, a relative who had come to this country earlier than her father, seeing how hard this girl was working and what a load she was carrying, took Minnie to the ballet on her birthday. Once it was *Giselle* and the other time *Swan Lake*. These were the only two times she had ever seen a ballet, but she was in love with it from the first moment. She remembered even now who the dancers were at those performances over fifty years ago and how they had danced each movement. Only one other person knew her secret, for she had never spoken to anyone of it since she was a child. In her tenement there lived a rich man. He was so rich that he took *The New York Times* every day! Whenever there was a ballet advertisement or review, he saved that page for her. In addition, whenever there were other newspapers in the trash bin, Minnie would look through them for anything related to the ballet. She told me that she especially used to look forward to the old *New York World* reviews.

This was clearly a serious matter. I had a friend who owed me a favor. She was a leading dancer in the Metropolitan Opera Corps de Ballet. I called her and asked her to spend an hour with a friend of mine in the hospital who was interested in ballet.

The next day Nina showed up at one o'clock. She said that she had a rehearsal at four-thirty but could spend an hour with Minnie. I introduced them and left them alone. When I came back in an hour, they were talking together so animatedly that they did not even see me. I returned at three, and they were still talking and this time they were holding hands. At four o'clock I came back and told Nina that I knew she was late and that I had a taxi downstairs with the motor running. As I walked her to the hospital elevator, Nina looked at me with amazement and said, "She knows more about the ballet than I do!" I went back to Minnie's room. She turned to me with stars in her eyes and said, "This has been the most wonderful afternoon of my whole life."

As one might imagine, Minnie and I talked a good deal about this experience and about the ballet and her feeling for it. Somewhere in our talk (I was never very clear from which one of us it came) arose the idea that Minnie was going to write a book about the history of ballet in New York City. There was never any talk of *publishing* a book; she really just wanted to write it.

I went to the public library and took out all the relevant books I could find. From hospital supply (and from all my friends' offices) I stole yellow pads, pens, and pencils. Minnie happily got to work.

And then it hit the fan. Suddenly I was in trouble. First the relatives. Her children descended on me in a fury. What was I trying to do with this illiterate old lady? Who did I think I was? Was I trying to give her "hope"? (I have never understood the meaning of this question, which has often been asked of me. Nor have I understood how and why hope and effort for the future are so often considered a sin.) The children went to the hospital clinical director and complained of "That charlatan who . . ." The clinical director listened gravely, said, "I'm glad that you brought this to me. I have had my eye on him for some time. Just leave it to me." He then promptly dropped the whole matter after he told me I obviously was doing very well!

The second group I was now in trouble with were the floor nurses. No longer was Minnie a "good" patient. Her bed, bedside table, and the floor under her bed were piled with yellow pads and books. When anyone attempted to move them or clean up, she screamed at them like a fishwife. When her meals were brought, she was usually too busy to eat and would gulp her food just before the tray was taken away. When they came to her to take her X ray or for some other procedure, she would tell them that she was right in the middle of something and that they would have to come back later. She often woke up in the middle of the night, turned on her light, and started writing "Because I just thought of something." No longer was she so sweetly agreeable on rounds. Instead of "Yes, doctor, I'm feeling much better today," it was much more likely to be "When am I going to be well enough to go home? I have a lot to do there and I want to go to the Metropolitan Museum to look at their collection of

Playbills. Let's improve the medication and get me out of here."
Everyone was angry with me for what I had done to this lovely
old lady.*

But—she began to gain weight. Her strength was increasing. This was before the days of CAT scans and so forth, and
so it was not possible to be very clear about what was happening
in her stomach, but by every sign we had, she was showing a new
and positive response to the medical program. She still needed
hospital care but certainly seemed to be getting better. Soon,
observing her physical improvement, the children got the pitch
and started to go to libraries themselves for books on ballet.
This relieved me of a good deal of work.

June was cold that year and so was July. Early in August a
heat wave hit. It was terribly hot and the hospital was not
air-conditioned. Further, it was on direct current and what air
conditioners could be bought were alternating current. (I spent
an afternoon downtown looking for a DC air conditioner for
the ward Minnie was in. I found one but it weighed a ton and
a half, and when I got it there the building engineer would not
let me have it brought into the building, saying the floors could
not hold it!) The average temperature on the floors was in the
high nineties all day and in the high eighties at night. We packed
patients in ice, transferred or discharged all we could, but many
had no better place we could send them. The patients on the
cancer service died like flies. In the charnel house the hospital
had become, Minnie died too.

---

*One of the signs I have used to tell how well I was doing with hospitalized
patients was how the floor nurses felt about my visits. As long as they seemed
glad to see me, I knew that the patient was still being "good" (as defined by
hospital standards) and therefore much less likely to get better. When the floor
nurses made it plain that they resented my coming, I knew that the patient
was becoming less concerned with the opinions and demands of others and
was becoming concerned with the growth of his or her own soul. I was making
progress! And the patient was fighting for his or her life! The recent studies
by Greer and associates have clearly shown that, statistically, "feisty" patients
survive their cancer diagnoses and medical procedures longer than do "accepting" or "apathetic" patients.

At the funeral, the oldest of her children described Minnie as a maple tree. All her life, he said, she had lived in muted colors, only just before she died had she blazed forth in reds, yellows, and orange. We were all very moved by this, but the most moving thing for me was that when I got back to my office, I found that one of her children had taped to my door a spray of maple leaves.

———————————

One of the most important parts of this method is the emphasis on individual approaches and solutions. If therapists encourage all people with cancer to seek a life-style that is uniquely theirs, *then the therapists must see the patients as individuals and treat them as such.* There is no one right way to relate to another human being (except for the general principle of doing as you would be done by), and each relationship is unique. It is crucially important for the therapist to exemplify this by his or her behavior and approach.

Further, no one explanatory system is valid for dealing with all patients. I was one of the lucky ones who was taught this early in my career. I had a marvelous undergraduate teacher in psychology—Richard Henneman—who taught us that there was no one way to look at human beings, that all systems limp, and that to understand what it means to be human needed a number of angles of approach. In Wittgenstein's terms, there is no one definitive photograph that we can make. We can, however, develop an album of sketches of a landscape that would help to illuminate the terrain. Henneman's course in the systems and theories of psychology was required for all psychology majors at the College of William and Mary, where I studied. Henneman started the course by teaching Behaviorism as if he were a devout Behaviorist. With zeal and fire he went through the first six weeks, and at the end of it, we were all convinced and dedicated Behaviorists. He then suddenly shifted and taught the next six weeks as a completely convinced Gestaltist. Then a period of Psychoanalysis, one of Stern's Personalism, and so on. At the end of the year we *knew* that there was value and truth in all of the systems, *that none had exclusive rights to the territory,* and that no one theoretical model could ever encompass the wonderful and complex thing that was a human being. We had learned that the wider our view, the more theoretical viewpoints we learned, the more sketches there were in our album, the more we could bring to our work as psychologists.

Years later I came to realize that the same lesson applied to psychotherapy: different patients were best worked with from different points of view, and no one therapeutic approach was useful for everyone who consulted me. During this period I attended a lecture at the Westchester Child Guidance Clinic. The speaker was a child psychiatrist named Annina Brandt, a lovely, zestful woman who must have been in her late seventies at the time. She talked with warmth and love of how it felt to be a child, of the long thoughts and sudden changes of mood, of the need for love, and of the often-incomprehensible perceptions of adults' activities. The staff, which was quite orthodox psychoanalytically, became more and more uncomfortable. Finally one of them interrupted her. "Dr. Brandt, what *school* do you belong to?" Brandt looked quite puzzled and hesitated. Finally she replied, "But how can I tell until I see the child?"

I recall the words of Dr. Joseph Michaels, a wise and experienced psychoanalyst, at a hospital staff conference. After the patient had been described by the physician working with him, brought in and interviewed in front of the staff, then had left, and the others had expressed their opinions, Michaels, Chief of the Service, announced his decision. He said: "This patient needs the Snarib Treatment and I want it instituted immediately." He then left the room. As no one there had ever heard of this treatment, we went in a body to the medical library. Intensive research failed to turn up a reference to it, to a Dr.

Snarib, or to anything else of relevance. The whole group then went to Michaels's office and one of us knocked on his door. He opened it, invited us in, and explained.

"I used this method so that you would all remember this lesson." (And it is over forty years and I still remember.) "Snarib is an acronym. It stands for 'Skillful Neglect and Rest in Bed.' That is what *this* patient needs. *He is a completely typical patient in that he is unique and what he needs is unique.* Anytime you find two patients who need exactly the same treatment, remember that the similarity is in your perception of them, not in them. And if you see more than two who need the identical treatment, it is quite likely that you are perceiving your own problem, not theirs, and prescribing for them what should be prescribed for you."

───────────────

Since then I have learned from my own experience that there are Freudian patients, Jungian patients, Existentialist patients, and all other varieties. There are patients I have been on a first-name basis with at the end of the first session, where it was "Joe," and "Larry," and there are patients with whom I have been on a formal, last-name basis after three years, where it was "Mr. Jones," and "Dr. LeShan," with a formal handshake at the beginning and end of sessions. Indeed, it is my belief that honest psychotherapists refer to other practitioners at least a third of the patients who come to them on the basis that the therapist is being hired to help the patient find the best for him or her and the best is a different therapist with a different personality.

As with Carol's case, I have found that it is important to be flexible in the time assigned for each session. For myself, there are some limits on session length. More than two hours at a time is too exhausting for me. I have, however, had patients for whom this was an ideal session length. I have also seen people for whom twenty-five minutes to a half hour were the best working times. I have varied session length between these two limits. Discussing this with patients at the beginning of the process, and at intervals along the way, makes for better work and also reinforces the basic lesson of the necessity of patients finding their own rhythms and style of life. Therapists who are not reasonably flexible and do not discuss session length reinforce the opposite lesson: that patients must adjust to the world rather than the reverse. Very often in our work we give contradictory messages. When we are forced to do so, it is absolutely necessary that the therapist be aware of this and communicate this awareness to the patient.

In a recent article in The New York Times on Memorial Sloan-Kettering Cancer Center, the author stated that researchers there are "still searching for agents that may activate the body's immune system against cancer."*

On the level that the search is being made at this research center—how molecules interact in the biological systems—no one knows the answers today. But on the level of human action—what should the individual with cancer do to mobilize his immune system and bring it to the aid of the medical program—we do know an answer. Unfortunately, this is not an answer that works every time to the desired degree, but it usually does have a very positive effect on the cancer-defense mechanism, one aspect of the immune system. It is also an answer that changes the tone and color of the individual's life in a positive direction whether or not he or she has cancer.

The method concerns people taking control over their own life—of searching for a life-style especially suited for them and, when found, actively working toward living this life.

For many individuals, this requires a complete restructuring of their thinking about themselves. A very large number of us grew up oriented toward what we should do rather than what we would enjoy doing; toward what we should want in our life

*"Dr. Mark's Crusade." The New York Times Magazine, April 26, 1987, p. 27.

rather than what we really want. Our actions are usually based on these "shoulds" rather than on the question of "what would fulfill me—what *style* of being, relating, creating would bring me to a life of zest?" This is the life, this life and the search for it, that mobilizes the immune system against cancer more than anything else we know today.

Zest and enthusiasm do not need to be expressed loudly and exuberantly. They come to us from living in the way we were built for, rather than our living in accordance with any special standards. One of the most zestful men I have ever known led a very subdued life. He was the comptroller of a medium-size private hospital. He loved his life and the quiet, rather solitary order it brought him. His happiest times would come toward the end of a fiscal year when the hospital books were off by something like seventeen cents out of a multimillion-dollar budget. Hank would arrive each morning, dressed in his neat three-piece suit, white shirt, and solid-color tie. He would go into his office, take off his jacket, and spend the day going over the hospital records day by day and transaction by transaction. At noon he would send out for a sandwich and coffee. His secretary handled most of the telephone calls during these periods, putting only the most important through to him. At the end of the day he would come out of his office fresh and calm, relaxed and smiling, get into his car and drive fifty miles home to dinner with his wife, then spend an hour listening to the radio and one studying ancient languages. Two evenings a week he worked as the unpaid business manager of an ecology organization. In the morning he would get up early, lift weights for an hour, and drive to work. On weekends he gardened in season, took long walks, and worked on his ancient languages. (When I knew him he was proficient in Latin, Greek, and medieval Italian, and was studying Middle English.) Such a life-style would have driven many of us (including me) insane within a very short period, but it suited him down to the ground. He had designed his life to suit his special structure and needs; he lived it quietly, fully, and with a great zest and enthusiasm that was not expressed outwardly but rather lived.

This concept of directing our lives from the needs of our individual structure rather than from what we believe we are supposed to be and do is so alien to many of us that often therapists must start small in retraining themselves and their patients to think and act in this way. What we as therapists are really saying is: "Do not worry about what the world wants of you. Worry about what makes you come alive because what the world *needs* is people who are more alive." Often, however, we must deliver this message in a wide variety of ways.

"Come now," we might say to a patient, "you have one day a week that is free of your need to make a living or to do your job. I want you to *plan* that day in advance. Plan it well. The goal is to give you the most memorable day, the *best* day for you that is possible. Plan that day and *follow* the plan."

If this is not psychologically possible for the person to do, the resistance to it is analyzed as in the older method of therapy. What is the unconscious statement that makes it impossible to do? (If therapists find they cannot do it themselves, then it is time for them to discuss and analyze this with their own control therapist, to shift their roles and become patients again while they analyze their own neurotic blockages in this area. Saying to someone else "Do as I say, not as I do" is a fruitless procedure.)

The anxieties produced by this procedure and the resistance to it are analyzed, but always in the *context* of their being part of the blocking forces that prevent people from achieving their own full life.

Or we might say something like this: "Your current program gives you two free evenings a week. At present they are being frittered away. They do not provide you with enjoyment, learning, or rest. Let us, in our imagination, look back from five years hence. What do you *wish* you had done with these evenings? I urge you to work on this question, find the answer, and carry it out. This is your assignment, which I hope you will accept for the next few months." Again, the fact that this is so hard to do for many individuals is examined in terms of the fact that it offers clues to why we stay so far away from our own best life.

Often the basic concept is so alien that we have to start even smaller. "I urge you," we might say, "to stop whatever you are doing a dozen times a day. Just pause to ask yourself one question: 'How do I feel about what I am doing right now?' Ask it seriously, *listen* inside for an answer, then go right on doing whatever it is. This will have two effects. It will teach you some things about yourself. It will also *retrain* you so that you begin to accept this as a serious question."

Sometimes the people will feel that the special life-style that is right for them requires a strong relationship with another human being. Without the other *one*—without Mr. or Ms. Right—they feel that they cannot function fully. As they do not have the other they believe they need, and have been unable to find him or her, the work seems hopeless, the goals unobtainable.

I have often dealt with this problem in a manner similar to the following: "Many times in my work here, people have said to me, 'How do I meet the other person I need? The singles' scene just doesn't work for me.' What they usually want is a *technique* to help them find the person of their dreams—that I should know of *this* place or *that* volunteer job or *that* cultural or interest group.

"Such techniques occasionally work, and whether or not they do, most people keep following them until they either (once in a while) succeed or just give up. There is, however, another approach that has far better results. Much more often it brings you together with a good other person for you, and even when it doesn't, it solves the problem.

"This other approach does not consist in searching for someone else but in making yourself into such an interesting person that others will come looking for you. It calls for turning around and approaching the problem from a completely different angle. You say, 'What can I do to make my life so interesting *to me* that others will want to share it? How can I make myself such a fascinating companion *to myself* that not only will others want to be near me, but I will be having such a good time that I don't care whether or not they appear? (After all, we all know that you get offered jobs and such when you do not need them!) How can I grow and garden myself so that I am having such a good time with my life, am enjoying myself so much that others will want to share the fun and even if they don't, I will still be having too interesting a time to worry about it?

" 'In this process, how can I be more and more *myself* so that others who would really like me if they got to know me would recognize who I am and therefore be attracted to me? How can I grow as such an interesting, unique, and *authentic* individual that others will be able to recognize me and respond? '

"The 'authentic' is important. Otherwise it will not work well. To the degree it does, the people you attract will soon find as they come closer that you are flying false flags and are far from what you are trying to appear to be. Relationships built on false premises soon collapse. Plato had a basic guideline for life that is very applicable today. It is 'Be what you wish to appear.' "

Therapists should never promise, either implicitly or explicitly, that the more people are their authentic selves—the more they respond in terms of who they really are and not in terms of the social "shoulds"—the more popular they will become with everyone. Being authentic will *not* make everyone like them; on the contrary, it will make people polarize around them, make others go to extremes. There are those—generally the ones you care most about—who will get more and more enthusiastic and say "Go, man, go!" or "Go, woman, go!" As these people see more and more who you really are, they will want to come closer and relate more intensively. Others, however, will have the opposite reaction. They will not like the particular kind of "corners" and "bones" that show in your personality. And the more you show them, the less they will like it.

"The only way to have everyone like you is to be so bland,

so homogenized, that no one has anything to dislike. Of course if you do this, no one will have anything to like either. No one likes or dislikes a custard: it just sits there and sogs at you. The more that you are yourself, the more people will go to extremes in their feeling about you. This includes those who will be attracted to you."

Franklin Roosevelt (who was elected President four times) understood this well. His favorite story about himself concerned the Westchester commuter who every day would come to the railroad station for his train, go over to the newspaper kiosk, put down his money, pick up *The New York Times*, glance at the front page, throw the paper back on the pile, and walk away. The newspaper vendor wondered about this for a long time. One day when the commuter's train was late, the newspaper vendor went over and asked him the reason for this repeated and strange behavior. "Oh," said the commuter, "I'm just interested in the obituaries." "But," was the reply, "you just look at the front page. The obituaries are on the back page." The commuter answered, "The son of a bitch *I'm* interested in—his obituary will be on the front page!"

No life-style is positively regarded by everyone. The more clear and articulated it is, the more people will go to extremes about it and about the person living it. However, the more people live the life that is right for them, the more they will be enjoying life and, as a general rule, the more the type of person that they would be attracted to will be attracted to them.

Sometimes people with cancer tell me that they want things to be as they were before the appearance of the illness. I call their attention to the fact that what people are depends on the interaction of two sets of factors—their genetic inheritance and their life experience. One of these aspects of their individual being has resulted in the appearance of a cancer. Genetic inheritance cannot be changed. With no change in the inner or outer life experience, we have the same two factors again interacting. Similar causes tend to produce similar results. To minimize the chances of a return of the illness we must change one of the two sets of factors. There is an old Chinese definition of insanity:

doing the same thing over and over again and expecting it to turn out differently.

"One of the hardest things," we might say to a patient, "is to escape from established doctrine. 'Common sense,' which Einstein once defined as 'that collection of prejudices which you have accumulated by age eighteen,' seems very strong as it tells us what we should want and strive for. It strongly indicates what we should try to be, what kind of personality we 'ought' to have, and this is reinforced over and over again by members of our peer group who, as they grew up, have picked up the same prejudices which we have.

"In order to examine this conventional wisdom further, it might be a good idea to look at what your peers seem to want out of life. You know them well. Make a list of what they want. What sort of life will they be living as they work for their goals, and what sort of life will they have when they have attained them?

"This is one of those exercises that do not work if you just do it in your head. It must be done with a pen and paper or a typewriter. When you've written down the list and descriptions, go over them with a different question. Are these goals that *you personally* want? Secretly, just between you and the paper, do you really want each one? The ways of life they lead to? Do you want those? Would you, living those lives, be glad to get up in the morning and be glad to go to bed at night? Underline in one color the ones you really want and in another color those you don't. Look at the color pattern. What have you learned about yourself? Write it down. What are *your* real goals? Your real *best* ways of life?"

If the process of self-examination and growth that I am describing is done during the course of psychotherapy, the past may have to be gone into as deeply as in more conventional psychotherapy. This is done, however, to analyze the blocks that keep the patient from being able to live out his or her true nature.

Individuals working alone will not explore and gain insight

to the same degree, but sometimes great progress *can* be made, life-styles can be changed greatly, and definite positive effects can be made on the immune system. A very large number of anecdotal cases in the cancer literature verifies this fact.

Many times these effects have been sufficient to halt or reverse the direction of growth of a serious neoplasm. Growth and change, like politics, are the art of the possible. We work on ourselves with the tools and materials that are both available and appropriate. A major factor—one that, as the philosophers say, is "necessary but not sufficient"*—is the *commitment* to grow and to change. This must be present, even if it is in the face of all our anxieties and fears. Depending on other factors, including many completely out of the person's control—such as genetic endowment, the stresses and supports perceived during early childhood, and so forth—it may then be possible to work effectively toward our own flowering. Sometimes it can be done alone. Sometimes it takes the help of a psychotherapist.

I often discussed the cancer-personality problem with a psychiatrist friend from Holland, Dr. Joost A. M. Meerloo. He had helped me develop an understanding of the problem. One day in the mid-1950s, I was sitting with him in his office when the bell rang. He asked me to stay and introduced me to the woman who came in. Together they told me the following story.

In the late 1940s, Ethel had consulted him professionally. She had a metastasized cancer of the breast and had been told that there was nothing further that could be done medically. Naturally she was frightened and upset and wanted some help in finding out how to live until she died. She explained that she had spent several sessions describing herself and her experiences, about how all her life she had wanted to travel on an ocean liner and see the world, but circumstances had never permitted this. Ethel had always felt that life on the sea would have been the ideal one for her and laughingly remarked that in a previous life she had probably been a sailor.

The best memories of her life had been before she had been

*That is, it is essential, but other things may also be needed.

married and in the first ten years afterward, when she had worked in an exclusive women's clothing store in Chicago. She had been a saleswoman and loved it. But even then Ethel had pored over travel brochures and dreamed of ships, cruises, and faraway places. Then had come the children and rich years as a mother and housewife. But her recollections of her earlier days were the richest she had.

Meerloo then pointed out that her husband was dead, her children lived on the other side of the continent and did not need her at the time (a matter that they had talked a good deal about), and that there was nothing to hold her back, no obligations or anyone else's needs that had to be taken into account. She was in no real pain or distress. Why didn't she travel *now*? The woman said, "But I'm sick. What could happen to me on a liner?"

Meerloo replied: "With the sickness you have, what could happen to you on the water that couldn't happen on land?

At that time the *Queen Mary* was making long, round-the-world cruises. Ethel took all her money (her oncologists had told her that she had a couple of months to live at the best) and invested it in a first-class cabin. Four months later she stormed into Meerloo's office and berated him, saying "Here I've spent all my money. I'm broke and I'm still alive!"

Meerloo said, "You would have preferred . . . ?" and they both broke out laughing. They talked awhile about how *at home* she had felt on an ocean liner and how natural and *right* being at sea had seemed to her. Meerloo had friends on the Holland-American Steamship Line and was able to arrange for her to get a job selling in a boutique on one of the liners. Since then, some eight years, when her ship was in port, she often called Meerloo and visited him. She loved her life and felt it was completely fulfilling. The breast cancer had shown no signs of increase since the middle of the first trip and had, she said, shrunk to about half its original size in the ensuing years. She had had no further medical treatment for it. Every year Ethel sent Meerloo (and her oncologist) a Christmas card, and after Meerloo died a few years later, she sent one for several years. I do not know what has happened to her after that.

3

CANCER AND
THE FAMILY

Harriet and Walter met in college where she was studying musicology and composition and he was studying painting, and fell in love. After the first month, neither had any doubt but that they would marry. In their senior year, they did and had their first child a year after graduation. They both wanted a family and decided that Harriet would give piano lessons and teach music in the local schools while Walter worked at becoming a painter. Ten years later they had three children, and he was selling his paintings regularly at a half dozen small galleries in Tucson, Phoenix, and Albuquerque. At the end of that time, she developed a lymphoma that spread rapidly and, in spite of all efforts, metastasized to several locations.

When I first talked with Harriet, everything in their lives seemed fulfilling and satisfying and I could find no trace of psychological factors. She kept telling me how fulfilling her work and her children were to her and what a wonderful relationship she had with her husband. Presently, however, discrepancies and clues began to appear. She had been very successful as a teacher, had more than a full schedule of private students and was turning away prospective pupils because of a lack of time. Two separate school districts, both adjoining the one she taught in, had asked her to teach for them also. She had composed a number of pieces for the local chamber music group, and they were constantly asking her for more and offering to send her scores to major orchestras or else make tapes for her to do so, but she "was just too busy and never got around to it." When I asked her how it could be that she was too busy to allow *them* to send the scores, she appeared to be confused and then angrily asked me, "How could *you* have any idea what it means to raise three children and support a family at the same time?"

She became, indeed, quite angry at me after I asked this question. I kept suggesting that she save her anger for the brief time necessary to answer the question to *her* satisfaction: "Why would it take her more time and energy to tell the chamber music group to go ahead and send the scores than it did to tell them not to?"

After a few minutes of glaring at me she became quietly thoughtful and then told me the answer she had known for a long time and never discussed with anyone. For over five years she had been aware that her talent was a first-rate one, and: "Walter's a wonderful guy and I love him more than anything, but as a painter he's strictly run-of-the-mill. He'll always make enough of a living to keep him in paints, brushes, and canvases, and that's about all. But his painting is so important to him that he will keep at it and enjoying his work and feeling good as long as he lives. And I'm not *ever* going to let that be taken away from him."

She had determined to keep her own talent hidden— "under a bushel basket" was the way she put it. Harriet felt that if she ever got recognition and Walter did not, it would destroy him, "and it would certainly end our marriage. He could never live with someone who made a real success while he hasn't. There would be too much constant reminder."

When I told her of the poet Auden's definition of cancer as "a foiled creative fire," she smiled sadly. I didn't know how to shake her evaluation of the situation. And perhaps she was right. After her death, the chamber music group collected all the pieces she had written, had them copied, and were prepared to send them off to several major orchestras. The husband said he would like to do this himself, and they gave him the copies. When I checked nine years later, they had still not been mailed out.

We in the helping arts are very much aware today that a person does not live alone, uninfluenced by anything in the present, but rather lives in a very real and dynamic context, usually that of a family or other intensively relating group. The days when psychotherapists could largely ignore this are thankfully long since gone. We know now that a very limited amount of time and energy is spent in the therapy room compared to the time and energy spent in interacting with the important others. Therefore, after a person is diagnosed as having cancer, it is of major importance that the family quickly becomes as positive a force for the patient's growth as it can be.

In the future, one or more of the new forms of family therapy may prove applicable to the cancer field. As I am not experienced or trained in any of these modalities, I cannot offer any serious conclusion about them. I can, however, describe my own experience in attempting to enlarge the area of positive stimulation of the patient's growth to include the family.

I have always attempted to weave the patient's most important "other" in as my ally in this work. Usually I would see the person alone, explain my approach and what I was attempting to do and why, answer any questions, and then try to enlist his or her aid. Among other things, I would usually say something like this:

"Right now we are in an emergency situation. Joe is the one who must grow and change as rapidly as possible. He is the one in the slot. But, if this marriage is to continue, *both* of you will probably have to change. It is most disruptive to a relationship when one grows and the other does not. *After Joe's turn, it will be yours.* During this first period one of the things for you to do is to begin to think about how *you* want to grow and change. What more do you want out of yourself, and what is the best way to work toward it? You should do some serious thinking about this now so that when your time comes you will be ready to move."

Of course sometimes both partners can actively work on their becoming at the same time. This is certainly best when it can be done. At worst, it usually makes for an interesting and stimulating time.

Usually both members of the pair readily accept the concept of the spouse (or significant other) as an ally in helping the person with cancer to find his or her own way. When the goal is that *both* must grow, the concept becomes even more widely acceptable. Only rarely does a spouse not cooperate in this. This generally occurs in marriages so toxic that both partners already know that its dissolution would be the best thing for them. Mostly, however, I have heard responses rather like the following:

"I've been telling Joe for years that if he hates his job so much, he should quit it. Do something else. We'll give up the maid and I'll go back to work. I'd much rather have a happy husband who didn't make so much money than a rich and dissatisfied one. But he never could seem to hear me when I said this."

This is the same Joe who has been telling me:

"I'd like to quit my job and get into real estate. But it would be a long grind and it would be a long time before I was making any real money. Mary grew up having the good things of life and needs them. I couldn't take them away from her."

Or, in a similar situation, Jane, who has cancer, says something like:

"I'd love to go back to work. I've always hated just being a housewife. It's the same jobs over and over again, and nothing ever really changes. But Tom likes a neat house and 'dinner on the table' when he comes home. These things are important to him and it's my job to see he gets them."

At the same time, Tom has been saying:

"If Jane really wants to go back to work—fine! It would be a new and interesting life for both of us. We can always eat TV dinners, they make them pretty good now, and they only take twenty minutes to get ready. I'll do my share of the shopping. I'd a lot rather have a wife who enjoyed her life and had interesting stories to tell about it than a neat house that gets dusted and vacuumed every day."

When possible, it is often advantageous for the spouse also to go into psychotherapy. The spouse's psychotherapist should be one *who understands and is sympathetic to* the type and model of therapy that the person with cancer is going through. It can be very disruptive to the marriage if the two partners are in therapies with different basic philosophies. Certainly when both are in therapy, the two psychotherapists should be in frequent communication, with the knowledge and consent of the patients.

One aspect of the family that *must* be taken into account when working with people with cancer is the children. If there is one generalization above all others that we can make about children—one statement that is almost universally valid—it is that they usually interpret important happenings in the family as being caused by something they did or by something they are. Further, children still believe that adults are freely able to decide on their own actions and their own destinies: after all, they can stay up as late as they wish and eat what they please! Therefore, if a parent becomes sick or dies, it is seen as caused in part by their feelings about the child. The basic statement, found at conscious or near-conscious levels of almost every child who had a parent die, is "If I were a better boy, Mommy would love me enough so that she would never leave me."

That it was the child's *fault* that a parent died is a short and almost inexorable step from this.

The universality of this belief and its importance for the child's future development cannot be overestimated. It *must* be taken into account. In dealing with it, an ounce of prevention is worth many pounds of cure. It should be dealt with at as early a stage of the parent's illness as possible. The books listed in the footnote* on this page should be in the office of every oncologist and of every therapist who works with people with cancer. The first, at least, should be read by every parent with cancer or by his or her spouse.

Even when children deny such beliefs, preventive work should still be done. One woman I worked with had a metastasized cancer and had had a leg amputated. I saw her at home. I had to come there between three and five in the afternoon. Before three there was no one else home and it was hard for her to get on her crutches and answer the door. After five several family members were there, and it was hard to work quietly. From three to five, however, her eight-year-old son was home from school. He would answer the bell and escort me to her room. After the session, I would go to his room, knock, and he would take me down to the entrance.

The mother was very ill and was slowly going downhill. She found it impossible to talk to the boy about this. The father had tried several times and each time just choked up and could not continue. No one else seemed able or willing to do it. Therefore one day, when the boy took me up to his mother's room, I asked him if, afterward, I could talk with him for a while. He said, "Yes, and I'll show you my trains." After duly approving the trains, I began to talk with him about how children sometimes

*E. LeShan, *When a Parent Is Very Sick* (Boston: Little, Brown, 1986), and E. LeShan, *Learning to Say Goodbye When a Parent Dies* (New York: The Macmillan Company, 1976).

feel when a mother is as sick as his was; how they blame themselves, and so on. He listened and then informed me that these
were very silly children and that he would never feel like that.
I told him I understood that *he* didn't feel that way, but that
many children . . . We talked in this vein for some time. Then
I told him I had to leave and suggested that on the next visit,
we could talk again. He replied: "Oh, yes, and you can tell me
more about those silly children and how they feel!"

When possible, the work with children is done by a parent,
relative, school nurse, minister, school counselor, or physician.
Sometimes, however, none of these is willing and able to do this.
It then may fall on a psychotherapist. Very often this work must
continue after a parent's death. I have had children come back
as grown-ups, fifteen or twenty years later, wanting to know and
to talk about the parent who died.

Once the psychotherapeutic relationship has started, it
goes without saying, I hope, that the therapist is *not permitted*
to stop the sessions with the patient or the survivors so long as
they are needed. Cancer often drains the family's financial resources. That they cannot pay any longer is not a reason to end
the work. After many years of seeing patients and their families
who worked with me as part of the hospital or clinic program
and at no extra expense to them, I can say with certainty that
the old saw that the patient must pay in order to benefit from
psychotherapy is complete nonsense. Payment is often necessary
for the sake of the therapist. It is not necessary for the sake of
the patient.

When possible, psychotherapy is done in a professional office.
In working with people with cancer, however, frequently this
is not possible and instead one sees patients in their homes or
in a long-term hospital room. Under these conditions, a cur-

ious, little-discussed aspect of psychotherapy becomes important.

There is something very special about a psychotherapy office. Confidentiality of what is said or experienced in it is assured. The room assumes something of the quality of a "magic circle." In it, people can explore feelings and then have control over how much is expressed outside of the office. People can examine and experience feelings in the comparative safety of the four walls and then have the control to *meter*, to censor as much as they wish, their expression outside.

In other locations, the situation is different. There is no magic-circle quality about the space within which patients work to free themselves. Exploration is therefore harder and slower.

One solution to this that can be very helpful is to encapsulate the session in time instead of in space—use some sort of brief, unobtrusive *ritual* at the beginning and end of each session to mark it off in time from the rest of the day. Often this can be something as simple as sitting in the same chair each time, placing a notebook, purse, or briefcase in the same place, and getting down to active work at that moment. The ending is also ritualized in a similar fashion.

In serious meditational exploration, the situation is the same except that the ritual is usually done by the person him-/or herself. A "centering" meditation (see Chapter 9) at the beginning and end of each session can serve as marks of separation. In both approaches, it is important that the same ritual be done regularly and, so far as is possible, without exception.

People working without either psychotherapy or a regular meditation program should follow a similar procedure. At least once a day, a period of time should be selected as their own. Here the basic statement is: "This time is mine. No one else's demands or needs are critical here. At this time, I try to get in touch with what I need, who I am, and what I want out of my life." The time should be marked off by a definite beginning and ending ritual.

Working with someone in a hospital room has its own peculiar difficulties. Unless the person has a room to him-/or herself, privacy can be a real problem. Sometimes this can be solved with a good deal of ingenuity and perhaps a good relationship with the nursing staff. Often they will know of a quiet corner where you can take a wheelchair for an hour. Yet sometimes even this is not possible. I have conducted long weeks of regular therapy sessions in a whisper that the person in the next bed could not hear through the drawn curtains. It is quite a strain, but sometimes it can be done!

Often completely unique solutions are needed. Marthe had started therapy in my office in the outpatient clinic where I worked. After a year she decided that she did not agree with the clinic's approach and left to continue at a more traditional treatment center. She wanted to continue psychotherapy with me, but she did not want to come to the clinic any more as she was embarrassed at seeing the staff there. She could drive a car but get around without it only in a wheelchair. She lived too far out in the suburbs for me to visit her very often. Twice a week, therefore, we would meet at 11:00 A.M. in the parking lot of the Metropolitan Museum of Art. Marthe would park her car and we would get out her wheelchair and get her into it. We would then get at the head of the line for the opening of the lovely cafeteria with its tables around the fountain. (Alas! This no longer exists.) As soon as the doors opened, she would go to our special table, which we had chosen because it had both privacy and a good view of the fountain. I would go to the serving tables and bring both trays to the table. We would eat, finish our coffee (the ending of which served as our opening ritual), and then have an hour psychotherapy session. At the end, I would signal the busboy to take our trays away (the closing ritual) and then, with me pushing her wheelchair, we would go through our favorite art galleries for a half hour. For both of us it was a good way to work, and it had the added advantage of our feeling refreshed by the paintings at the end.

It was a unique approach that fitted the situation and our personalities. The last is important. If it had not fitted us to work in this way, it would not have been a viable procedure. Freud may well, as the story goes, have treated Mahler successfully while they both rode horseback. It apparently fitted both their personalities. It would definitely not have fitted those of Marthe and myself.

■

The stress of cancer may in one family bring about much fuller and deeper communication between the members and in another family have the opposite effect. It is an important task for those family members involved to keep a careful eye on the effect the diagnosis and the disease have had on their ability to communicate with one another. Where communication has not been increased, they should make conscious efforts to deepen it and make sure that it is open on crucial issues. The key word is often *respect*. Family members must have respect for one another. We shield someone from the truth in most cases because we do *not* respect their strength and their ability to handle the truth. Treating other adult members of the family as if they were children does not increase their ability or the family's ability to deal with a crisis.

If the family members cannot keep their lines of communication open, it is the task of close friends or of professionals to do this. Fortunately, for example, it is not as common as it used to be for the medical professional to hide the truth of a diagnosis from the patient. Sometimes, however, the diagnosis is not hidden but rather softened. Recently a man I knew had an exploratory study. The diagnosis was a malignant cancer, and the man's wife was told this, that it was a dangerous cancer, and that they needed to remove his urethra, one kidney, and part of the bladder. The man, however, was told that it was a benign tumor and that they wanted to remove these organs for prophylactic purposes. The wife checked with her own physician who talked to the oncologist and confirmed to her what she had heard. She then told her husband so that he could decide on the course of treatment on the basis of accurate information. When I talked with him the next day, he seemed quiet and determined. He told me that he had been a merchant marine officer for many years and one thing that he had learned for certain was that it was far more dangerous not to know what the situation was than to know about it, however bad it might be. "I'm never really afraid of anything I know about. I can decide what to do and do my best. It's the things I don't understand that frighten me. I don't know how to act or what to do." This was a strong man who could face what he had to if given as much information as possible.

That afternoon, however, when he spoke to his physician, the physician denied what the wife had said, saying it was "only a tumor that we are taking out so that we don't have any more trouble in this area." The man was furious with his wife for frightening him so. The children also angrily reproached her. Ultimately the man's religious leader, after talking to the oncologist, had to talk to the man, his wife, and the children all at once and clarify the whole story. The patient then began to take control of the situation, getting another surgical consultation, asking about possible alternative programs of chemotherapy and radiation and the statistics on each of them. Finally he decided on a straight chemotherapy program and went through it. So far the effects seem to have been positive and the cancer no longer is visible on CAT scans.

In dealing with the family, psychotherapists and others must keep in mind that there are two separate kinds of denial. The healthy kind is analogous to how the body treats a simple flesh wound. Until the healing process is well advanced, the body forms a scab over the wound to protect it. This is a positive procedure, and when the healing has taken place the scab drops away. Very often after a diagnosis has been given, the person is reeling from the shock and is not ready to deal with it. Denial can be the healthy protective scab formed over the wound.

The second kind of denial persists for a long period and weakens patients' relationships (and therefore their resources to deal with the problem) and prevents them from taking responsible action. This is the unhealthy kind of denial.

Denial may be either conscious (usually adopted in order to protect someone else) or else unconscious, where the person actually believes it. In either case a denial is accepted and not moved against unless there is a good reason. No one has a right to attack the person's defenses under these conditions unless they are seriously interfering with his or her life or ability to deal with the illness.

One man told me: "This is a good hospital. Not like the last one I was in." When I asked him what the differences were, he said: "In the last place they told me I had cancer. Here they are treating my arthritis and I'm getting better." Clearly, here I accepted such denial without argument, as one would in the case of the surgeon I saw who was a patient on the oncology service of the hospital in which he had operated for many years. He had had surgery and radiation and told me of the "disseminated arthritis" that was causing him so much pain and suffering. The message was clear and there was no reason to disagree with his diagnosis.

It is quite a different matter where the denial is maintained for the sake of others and/or where it interferes with the person's access to his or her own source of strength or ability to deal with the current life problems. I recall one afternoon that was typical of so many during the years I worked on the cancer service of Trafalgar Hospital in New York City. In the bed was a sixty-seven-year-old man with a severe colon cancer. Next to the bed was his wife of forty-one years holding his hand. They both talked of his "bowel obstruction," which was being dried up, they said, by radiation. They both knew the diagnosis (as I had learned by talking privately to both of them), but publicly denied it. She at the doctor's suggestion and he taking the cue from her and from his physician denied it to each other in order to "spare" the other. These two people had an excellent marriage and had over the years been a source of support and help to each other. As they could not talk about the biggest thing in the room and in the world and could not talk very much about anything else because of where it might lead (after all, talking about last year's vacation could lead to talk about future vacations and so forth), they were soon reduced to discussing only the trivial: weather, television programs, and sports news. They could communicate only about things that had no consequences. They sat close together physically, loving and needing each other, yet separated by a glass wall of deceit, fear, and pain that stretched from wall to wall and floor to ceiling. His main source of strength was cut off as was their mutual ability to deal realistically with the problems.

As no one else was available to do the needed job, I came into the room and spoke approximately as follows: "Let us be honest with each other. You two people love and need each other and are kept apart by trying to protect the person you love most. This protection really has the opposite effect; you both are weaker and more alone and frightened because of it. We all know it's cancer and we are all frightened. No one is giving up hope. There are the tools and methods we are now using, and if these fail, although we wouldn't use them unless there was a very good chance they would work and if we didn't expect them to work, there are more available and more being invented every day. But it's a *scary* situation, and you two deal better with things when you are working together than when you each are alone. I'll be outside if you need me."

I then stepped outside the door and waited in the corridor (with my shirt soaking wet from *my* compassion and anxiety about how I was dealing with this profoundly human and moving crisis), because I knew that after a little time alone to share what they had been going through, they would need me to answer questions or to find out how to find the answers themselves.

In deep stress, when under the hammer of fate, many people do far better if they are in real and authentic communication with those they love. Where this has been weakened or stopped, it is the task of those most deeply involved—the patient, the spouse, the most important "other," the professional—to do what can be done to repair and strengthen the relationship. Most people can handle the tremendous stress, pain, and confusion of a cancer diagnosis better when they are working and crying together than they can when they are each alone.

4

HOW TO SURVIVE
IN A HOSPITAL

Overheard in a hospital corridor:

> FIRST WOMAN: The doctor said she should take the medi-
> cine regularly.
> SECOND WOMAN: Doctors, what do they care?

> VISITOR: How do you like the people in this hospital?
> HOSPITAL PATIENT: There are no people here. There are only
> doctors, nurses, and patients.

These two true incidents have in their implications a
strange grain of truth. When you enter a hospital, you are
entering a new world. If you understand this, you will know
better how to behave and how to achieve the maximum possible
benefits from your stay. You will also know how to avoid the
special pitfalls and dangers implicit in being a hospital patient.

First you must understand what a hospital *is*. It is a business
organization, in the last analysis, run by accountants, which sells
certain tests, remedies, and procedures related to disease. It is

staffed by people who came into the field generally from the best of motives. They were given a medical education and are in a medical system oriented to viewing the patient not as a person but as a broken machine. They work in a milieu that reinforces this orientation by ghettoizing the patients, segregating them by disease or dysfunctioning organ system. Because the staff stays in the hospital and patients come and go, they eventually begin more and more to see the hospital procedures as something that should be designed for their own comfort and convenience rather than for the patients'. Patients in pain, anguish, and fear constantly pressure them to behave in omniscient and omnipotent ways. Little by little they begin to act as if they could fill these roles, and train younger colleagues also to act in this way. Presently they begin to believe that these are their proper roles and become upset when challenged.

Many doctors are so completely oriented to fighting disease and ignoring the sick person that, in catastrophic illness, they often seem to be asking themselves: "How many heroic measures and mutilating operations can be charged to the patient (or to the insurance company) before death—the final method of consumer resistance—is allowed to intervene?"

They define a *good* patient as one who accepts their statements and their actions uncritically and unquestioningly. A *bad* patient is one who asks questions to which they do not have the answers, raises problems with which they are uncomfortable, and does not accept hospital procedures as necessarily wise, useful, or intelligent. There is a tremendous pressure on the staff to regard the institution's rules as correct and the individual patient who objects to them as wrong. In spite of all these pressures, an amazingly large minority of the staff at most hospitals do care about their patients and regard them as individuals. Yet a majority succumb to a greater or lesser degree to the pressures and become institution- rather than patient-oriented.

The high cost of medical care arises in large part from duplication of services among neighboring hospitals, which is largely a result of competition for prestige (and profits). If patient care were the major concern, it would be easy for the boards of directors of neighboring hospitals to come to an agreement about which hospitals should specialize in which services. As specialized equipment and facilities are becoming increasingly expensive, this kind of agreement would save a great deal of money. However, realistically, asking hospitals to do this is roughly the equivalent of asking Ford and General Motors to agree about which one will make small cars and which one will make station wagons.

For even the most dedicated physician or nurse, it is very difficult to maintain a service orientation while working in an institution devoted to profit making. It soon becomes clear to all employees that the product of their organization is tests and medical procedures, not patient care. The attitude that "the care of the patient comes first" is difficult to maintain when the entire hospital has another attitude entirely. What is amazing about modern hospitals is that there are so many caring people working in them and that the patient care is as good as it is.

If you recognize that hospitals are businesses selling a product and that they are a part (with the insurance companies and the pharmaceutical houses) of one of the largest and most lucrative industries in the United States, you will not be too surprised at some of the incidents of complete "uncaring" that you will probably encounter during any reasonably long stay in a hospital. Within just a few weeks' time, I have personally seen the following:

1. A postsurgical patient was returned to his bed, but his nurse's bell was not attached. He was the only patient in a multiple-bed room. No one else entered the room for six hours. Part of this time he was in severe pain and unable to summon help.

2. A patient unable to move by himself was left on a bedpan for two and a half hours. No one answered his bellpull, and his back muscles became knotted in pain. Finally, another patient passing in the hall heard him weeping, asked him what the problem was, and then went to the nurses' station at the end

of the hall, where he convinced a nurse's aide that she ought to respond to the patient's agony.

3. A patient who had returned from major abdominal surgery two days before had just had her catheter removed after voiding a large quantity of urine. She was now, an hour later, in extreme pain, her muscles spasming and threatening to tear open her incision. The patient complained that she had to void more urine. For over an hour three different nurses told her that she was hysterical. She was given tranquilizers and told that she was making a nuisance of herself, and that there were patients who had *real* pain and needed the nurses' attention. Suddenly, in the midst of her crying it became apparent that she was wetting the bed. The nurses looked at the wet sheets and decided to put the catheter back. When it was in, she voided 700 cubic centimeters of urine (that's a lot) through it. Not one of the nurses apologized or indicated in any way that they had been brutalizing the patient.

I could mention many more incidents of this kind that I have witnessed, but those cited give a sense of what may well happen during any hospital stay. I should add that these three incidents happened to intelligent, middle-class patients in hospitals with international reputations. It is because of incidents such as these, as well as other more serious mistakes that can have long-range effects, that you need to know how to defend yourself in a hospital.

During the same period of time that I saw these unfortunate events, I saw a much larger number of examples of caring, protective, and lifesaving behavior.

When you enter a hospital for a procedure or set of procedures, you are immediately subject to a routine whose effect is to strip you of all signs and symbols of your autonomous adult status and make you into a passive, dependent, childlike person who will not question or oppose those in authority. You can no longer decide what you will wear or eat, or go anywhere alone (often not even to the bathroom). Strangers take complete authority over your life and destiny, order you to wake up, go to sleep, turn over to be examined or washed, and generally act as if you are a not-too-bright child and they are adults.

Hospital patients are made to follow passively a routine, which they are prevented from comprehending by a strange and esoteric language and by the attitude that they simply do not have the training or knowledge to understand what is happening. They are quickly made to feel that a "good patient" behaves in the same way as a good and obedient child, who does as he is told, never asks difficult questions, and agrees that everything is fine as long as the adults are in charge (no matter what the actual situation is).

A friend, whom I admire greatly, was hospitalized after a heart attack. While in the cardiac care unit, she was attached to a machine that monitored her heart. Suddenly the machine stopped clicking away. A nurse came galloping into the room and was about to do various dramatic things to start my friend's heart pumping again, when my friend pointed out sharply that she was sitting up in bed, drinking some orange juice, and was very much alive. The nurse shouted, "But you *can't* be! Your heart has stopped beating!" My friend suggested that maybe the *machine* was the problem, an idea that seemed to strike the nurse as ridiculous. But shortly thereafter an electrician arrived on the scene.

I think my friend's story is a realistic metaphor for what life is like in many hospitals these days. There are very many exceptions, thank heavens, but the age of technology has turned some hospitals into machine shops in which advanced and lifesaving equipment is looked up to with awe, whereas people are considered an incidental inconvenience.

When you are desperately ill and realize that doctors and machinery and hospital care may well make the difference between life and death, your own judgment and your sense of personal identity are often impaired. Think how many weak and sick and frightened patients there are who might almost have been convinced that they *were* dead when the machine stopped working!

In his excellent book *Coping with the Crises of Your Life,*

Edgar Jackson, probably the world's outstanding specialist in crisis management, describes very well what happens when one becomes a hospital patient. Even a professional who knows the hospital procedures and routines is quickly and expertly reduced from an independent adult to a passive child.

> From that moment on, I was no longer the person I had been. Instead, I was a pliable, compliant inhabitant of a world of vague feelings and limited comprehension. I had been delivered, body, mind, and spirit, into the hands of my physicians. I was a completely dependent and defenseless creature surrounded by those who exerted authority over me.

Doctors often defend the process of patient infantilization by insisting that it is necessary for the smooth running of the hospital, is what is wanted by the patients, and, in fact, is good for them. The infantilization is, of course, simply for the convenience and emotional comfort of the staff, not the patients, and is a product of the basic belief that people who are sick are like machines that are broken. They don't work (that is, can't function as adults) and therefore must be fixed by a mechanic. Naturally, the machine sits there completely passively while the mechanic does all the work. The staff has been trained to deal with diseases and not with people. And this is what they do.

Max Parrott, president of the American Medical Association, wrote:

> It has often been said that the technical aspects of medicine are easy. The difficult part is dealing with the personality of the patient, the so-called psychological or human factor. This takes up a great deal of the time of the practicing physician. It is harder on the doctor's constitution than all of the technical aspects of medicine. It may even cause his or her demise, in the case of a physician with an autonomic nervous system that can't take the heat.*

---

*Quoted in Irving Oyle, *The New American Medical Show* (Santa Cruz, Calif.: Unity Press, 1979), p. 25.

Some years ago I instituted a program in a hospital with many long-term patients. An hour after each patient was admitted, a volunteer wheeled into the patient's room a cart containing a hundred good-size reproductions of famous paintings. The reproductions were professionally mounted on light beaverboard and the patient was invited to make a selection and decorate his or her room. The volunteer returned once a week to ask the patient if he or she wanted to exchange the prints for others. The program cost the hospital nothing, except for the time of one volunteer. (The paintings were donated by an art company to which I had explained the purpose.) Yet it was instituted against the strong opposition of most of the staff. The only objection verbalized was that the program "would cause confusion." The unspoken objection was that it would give a patient a sense of individuality, of being a person with a disease, rather than being a disease with a person somehow attached to it, and that it treated the patients as adults. Patient response to the program was very strong and positive, and the program continued very successfully for two years. Within three months of my leaving the hospital for another job, the program was discontinued.

Another example would be the experience of anyone who has battled with hospital personnel to establish a simple rule: nonmedical personnel such as floor sweepers, newspaper sellers, and so forth should be required to knock at a closed hospital room door (behind which someone might be sitting on a bedpan) before entering the room. The staff's fierce and emotional opposition to such a rule reveals their basic attitude that the patient is no longer an individual human being worthy of respect.

We know from long experience that treating patients as individuals and expanding their sense of themselves as individuals and adults serve to mobilize their self-healing abilities and bring them to the aid of the medical program. (Every experienced oncologist knows, for example, that "bad patients" tend to survive longer and to respond better to medical intervention than do "good patients.") However, along with the basic orientation that sick patients should be seen only in terms of their disease and that all results are a product of the formal medical intervention and not the individual's self-healing powers, this information is ignored; the average hospital's antitherapeutic routine weakens patients' ability to fight for their own recovery.

The concepts of self-defense and self-repair are central contributions of holistic medicine. The idea—not new to medicine, but one that has, in this century, played only a minor role—is that if given a positive environment—socially, emotionally, nutritionally, spiritually—the body's self-healing abilities can do a great deal. This is in accord with the famous statement of the great physician Harvey Cushing: "The task of the physician is to protect the patient from the patient's relatives so that nature can heal him." We are just beginning to appreciate the wisdom behind the wit of this statement and to find out all the things we have to protect the patient from. Sadly, these often include our own medical techniques.

When you enter a hospital, it is important for you, or someone with you, to understand the medical situation. You have left the private relationship with your physician and entered a large organization devoted to selling a product and making a profit. Although the hospital is staffed by many people, most of them caring and concerned about you, the overall organization is dedicated, as are *all* organizations, primarily to perpetuating its own existence and growth.

For this new situation you need to prepare a plan.

First, particularly if the procedures are going to be strenuous or will include surgery, if possible have a friend or relative who can be your advocate. Preferably this person should be someone who is not likely to be easily overawed and is not afraid to make a fuss and to ask difficult questions. Not being cut off from the outside world, not being stressed by pain, illness, or surgical procedures, this advocate can represent you when and if you are unable to represent yourself. By and large, the more interest your relative or advocate shows in your health, the better hospital care you will get.

A few years ago I was visiting a close relative in one of

Manhattan's finest hospitals. She was in a double room. The woman in the next bed was in her late seventies, very weak, and obviously malnourished. Each time I saw her, she seemed thinner and more like a refugee from a Nazi concentration camp. One day I saw her lunch tray being picked up and returned to the cart after lunch. The tray was untouched. She had eaten nothing. I made it my business to be there at dinner the following day. The same thing happened. Her tray was brought to her, set on the bed table in front of her, and an hour later was picked up and taken away. She was too weak and malnourished to eat.

Deciding to be her advocate, I went to the charge nurse on the floor and reported the situation. She promised to take care of it. However, at lunch the next day nothing had changed. I then went downstairs to the nursing supervisor's office and again fully reported the story. By that evening there was dramatic improvement. A nurse's aide had been assigned to the woman at each meal. The patient quickly started to gain weight and strength and by the time my relative left the hospital, she was eating by herself, walking up and down the corridor, and was at least ten pounds heavier.

If I had known her physician, I would certainly have reported the problem to him or her before telling the charge nurse. If I had had no success with the nursing supervisor's office, I would have gone to the office of the administrative director. For personal care the chain of complaint is: physician, charge nurse, nursing supervisor, hospital administrator, hospital director.

Once you have an advocate, your second priority is information. Before you enter the hospital, there are certain facts you should have and certain questions you should ask.

1. Who is the physician in overall charge of you? Make sure that there is someone who is running the show who has an overview of you and the problem that brought you to the hospital. Ideally that person should be your personal physician and, in most cases, it will be. But be certain that this is the case, and find out how often you will see him or her before you enter the hospital.

Unless there is a coordinating physician, very often in the modern hospital a diagnosis is made according to the specialty of the diagnostician rather than to the illness of the patient. For example, a patient who sees a psychiatrist may receive a diagnosis of "psychosomatic gastrointestinal disorder," whereas if he sees an internist, the diagnosis may be "pylorospasm." In one case the problem is seen as in the mind, in the other case in the gut. In neither case is there likely to be a multilevel approach to treating the entire person and the many factors that contribute to the disease.

2. What is the diagnosis, and how certain of it is your physician?

3. What is the usual course of the disease, both with and without therapy?

4. What are the side effects of the therapy?

5. What alternatives exist?

When diagnostic tests are prescribed, you will want to know how painful they will be, what side effects they will have, and—most important—whether they will make a real difference (a *real difference* is a difference that *makes* a difference). Will the physician's course of action change depending on the results of the test? *If not, there is no reason to take it.* There is an increasing tendency to give more and more tests. Between 1967 and 1972, for example, the number of laboratory tests conducted per hospital admission increased 33 percent. But there was no corresponding increase in medical knowledge during that period.

Remember that the hospital is in the business of selling services, and these include diagnostic tests. In addition, no physician or hospital was ever sued for malpractice for making too many tests and being *too* thorough in an examination.

Some medical students were asked why they wanted to do a particular arduous diagnostic procedure on their patient. One of them answered that their chief resident had said that only three things were important in medicine: "The diagnosis, the diagnosis, and the diagnosis." While the story may be apocryphal, it illustrates a common medical attitude, especially in the idealized setting represented by the university teaching hospital. The search for a diagnosis may acquire a life of its own, and in working toward that diagnosis the patient's original complaints, life situation, needs, fears, and economics may become irrelevant. The scenario is directed more by available technology, the special interests of the hospital personnel, the schedules of the institution, and above all, the hidden nature of the disease, which must be found because, like Mount Everest, "it is there."

The more tests that are performed, the more likely the results of at least one will look unusual. Tests generate more tests, and test results often lead to unwanted and unnecessary treatments. As patients, we then find ourselves embarked on a medical program we do not need.

The famous Wassermann diagnostic blood test for syphilis has been used for forty years. Only lately have we discovered that it is a hypersensitive test and that about half of the individuals diagnosed as syphilitic by it *did not have the disease!* Numerous other medical procedures are more popular than validated.

There is often a deep gap in the communication between patient and physician. They may seem to be communicating and think that they are, but their assumptions are so different that both are bound to be disappointed and angered by their relationship.

Often the patient is saying something like: "Make me feel

good. Fix my life, which isn't working. That is what I am paying you for."

While the physician is saying something like: "Respect me, because I bring the best of modern science to the treatment of your disease. That is what you are paying me for."

Neither is really aware of his underlying assumptions. Neither is going to be happy with the results.

One study showed that when a physician said to a patient, "You will be going home in a few days," most patients thought this meant one or two days. Yet to a majority of the physicians, it meant two to four days. Communication is a fragile thing at best. When you are speaking to a physician about an illness, keep checking to make sure that you are hearing each other. Many problems can be prevented if you take it upon yourself to keep the lines of communication clear. Your advocate may be helpful here.

Do not let yourself be ignored if there is something that the physician should know or should be paying attention to. The word *no* is powerful. Use it and be stubborn in repeating it until you are convinced that your objections have been responded to reasonably. Recently a patient was being evaluated in a large New York hospital. Although it was not urgently indicated, and was not of very high priority in the examination, the physician decided to use a dye test (IVP) for evaluating kidney function. The patient told the doctor that she was allergic to the dye, that on a previous examination in another city she had been given the test and had had a severe negative reaction. Because this reaction was not in the physician's experience, he did not listen to her and gave her the test anyway. The patient died. A simple but stubborn "No, I will not take the test" would have saved her life. Occasionally you will also have to shout and throw things to get the hospital staff to pay attention to you as a specific individual. You are very likely, of course, to get angry reactions if you say no to something, but your stand may well save your life.

You must also control the number of people who will give you physical examinations. The resident on your service needs to examine you because if anything goes wrong, he or she has to make quick decisions and so must know your body from direct examination. Ask your personal physician if there are any other physicians who *must* do this. If there are, list them on a pad of paper on your bed table and refuse anyone else. You are allowed to say no. When you are ill there is no reason that you should cooperate in a hospital research project or help an intern build up his or her quota of examinations by doing one on you.

If you are a woman, only one person should do a breast examination. Unless you are in a gynecological service, no one should do a pelvic examination, and you do not need a Pap test. If your physician wants to make an exception to these particular rules, he or she should explain the reasons in detail. "Hospital procedure" is not a reason.

On the pad of paper on your bedside table, have your physician list all the medications you are supposed to get, at what times you get each, and *what each one looks like.* If a nurse or aide gives you a medicine that doesn't fit your physician's description, refuse it. Even at the best hospitals, a lot of medications get sent to the wrong people.

Find out what diet you will be on and whether you can have food brought in from the outside. As Hippocrates said, "Food or drink slightly inferior in itself, but more pleasant, should be preferred to that better in itself but less pleasant."

You can, of course, go to either extreme on this. The rule of some nutritionists has been that food should be "good of itself," pure and free from contaminants, even if it tastes like parsnip sprouts in wallpaper glue. The other extreme is that the appetizing quality of food—the way it looks and tastes—should be the critical factor and it does not matter very much if the food is full of the kinds of additives that otherwise are used in the manufacture of tanning materials. Both cases imply that some aspects of the human being are of real importance and certain other aspects are not. From the viewpoint of serious holistic medicine, *all* aspects are of real importance, although a health specialist may, of necessity, work first with one aspect and later with the others. In regard to food, Hippocrates was clearly suggesting a middle course, in line with our modern viewpoint, with the emphasis slightly on the appealing quality.

The average hospital serves food that is neither appetizing nor nutritious. Hospitals have generally managed to produce food that is "inferior in itself"—white bread is usually served along with nearly everything else full of contaminants—and at the same time unappealing and unappetizing. They have managed to combine the worst features of institutional food and junk food. Yet a few hospitals, employing trained chefs and nutritionists, have shown that it is just as possible to produce attractive and healthful meals.

The most important people involved in your personal care are the nurses. The charge nurse (the chief nurse of your floor) on each of the three shifts will come in to introduce herself and to see you the first day. If she does not, send her a message that you would like to meet her. One of the supervisors of the nursing service will also look in every day or so. The charge nurse and the nursing supervisor are the ones to talk to if there is any problem with personal care. Feel free to complain. You do not have to be a good child. Complaints *will* get you better service.

In 1972 the American Hospital Association adopted a series of resolutions for patients' protection. These became known as the Patient's Bill of Rights. It is now accepted by all hospitals sanctioned by the Joint Commission on Accreditation of Hospitals (JCAH). The Bill of Rights states in part:

Any competent adult has the absolute right to refuse treatment. Any competent adult has the absolute right to refuse to be examined by any particular individual. Any competent adult has the absolute right to refuse to participate in teaching activities.

You also have the right to know the results of all tests made on you, including your blood pressure and pulse rates. It will make it easier, and save a lot of arguments, if you tell your physician to make a note in your chart and to inform the nursing station that any questions you ask are to be answered.

Hospital personnel use all sorts of excuses, but the real reason they tell patients as little as possible ("Hush, dear, everything is fine") is because patients are supposed to be good children who don't ask questions, but do just as they are told.

You also have a right to see your chart any time you wish. (Most hospital personnel become terribly upset if you ask to do this, but a lawyer will bear you out and if necessary remind the hospital that you are an adult, competent human being who retains a lawyer.) There is, however, one problem with this. It may *not* be wise to read your own chart. Very often certain terms have one meaning for the layperson and quite another for those with formal medical training. There may be material in your chart that appears alarming to you but is not at all alarming to the physician. My advice is to ask your physician to keep you closely informed of test results and the other material in your chart, but don't try to read the chart yourself. If, however, you cannot get the information verbally, read it.

You can leave the hospital at any time. If anyone prevents you from doing so, you can sue for false imprisonment. The hospital may request you to sign an against-medical-advice (AMA) form, but they can only request this and cannot hold you if you refuse. Incidentally, studies done on patients who left hospitals against medical advice show that few later regret it, and few experience adverse effects (about 5 percent for each). The main damage done is usually to the hospital staff's sense of omnipotence.

Unauthorized medical treatments (except in clear and obvious life-or-death situations) constitute assault and battery. It does not matter whether the treatment was advisable or not, successful or not. Consent is the key.

As far as surgical procedures go, the rule is the less the better. Do not allow surgeons to remove organs "because there might be trouble with them later and as long as you're opened up, you might as well eliminate the potential problem. . . ." A large number of women with fibroid cysts of the uterus have had their uterus and ovaries removed on this basis. The surgeons told them that they could always use synthetic hormones. Then it was found that the use of synthetic hormones tended to produce cancer. That treatment is now unavailable. I know of not a single surgeon who ever expressed any regret over these women or apologized to one of them.

In contemplating the removal of an organ or organs, remember that Nature does not indulge in luxuries. As Galen wrote: "Nature does nothing in vain." If it is there, there is a good reason for it. No substitute is going to be as good (Mother Nature knows best). An organ should be removed if the alternative *at this time* is completely unacceptable. You can always have it removed later. You can't have it put back.

No one seems to have been disturbed that after recent doctors' and hospital strikes in a number of cities (during some only 15 percent of the city's hospital beds were used), there was no noticeable increase in suffering, and certainly no increase in the mortality statistics. A strike in a factory that reduced its usage to 15 percent of normal would certainly lead to a decline in the goods produced. If the product of the hospital is supposed to be a decrease in suffering and a lowering of the death rate, why do we not see evidence of this? Perhaps we have no adequate measure of human suffering. But we do know how many people die each month and of what. Is it possible that there is far more wrong with our medical and hospital system than we've dreamed? Is this why no one has asked if the other 85 percent of the hospital beds is really necessary, or simply connected to a very large business that has lost sight of some of its primary goals—such as caring for the suffering—and now operates largely in terms of profit and loss? Is the reason we do not inquire about this other 85 percent of the hospital beds the same reason that no one asks why General Motors can't start making fewer cars each year?

In 1934 the American Child Health Association studied doctors' reports on the advisability of tonsillectomy for 1,000 children: 611 had already had their tonsils removed; the remaining 389 were then examined by other physicians and 174 more were selected for tonsillectomy; this left 215 children whose tonsils were apparently normal. Another group of doctors were put to work examining these 215 children, and 99 of them were adjudged in need of tonsillectomy. Still another group of doctors was then employed to examine the remaining 116 children, and nearly half were recommended for the operation.

Among the things you should carry with you to the hospital are the usual medications you take regularly or occasionally (such as headache or allergy remedies). Ask your regular physician *before you enter the hospital* if any of these are contraindicated by the procedures you will undergo. Then keep your medications in your purse or bedside table. If someone tries to take them away, you or your advocate friend should simply forbid it. Just because there are "hospital regulations" doesn't mean you have to obey them. In addition, particularly if you are to have surgery, bring some glycerine suppositories. People are frequently badly constipated after surgery and by many tests, and by many painkillers. For reasons I don't understand, most hospitals will give you a suppository only when you are impacted up to the shoulder blades.

On the aforementioned pad, write your personal physician's office and home telephone numbers as well as the name and numbers of any physicians who will have much to do with you while you are a patient—surgeon, anesthetist, and the like. Use any and all these numbers if you need to.

When you are in the hospital with a serious condition, there is, unfortunately, one other thing of which you must be aware. In many hospitals psychiatrists and psychologists are seen as special disciplinary arms of the medical service. If you ask too many questions, or—horrors above—decide against a procedure that the hospital thinks is right for you, the medical staff is likely to ask for a psychiatrist to visit you. The rationale behind this is that if you disagree with the decision that you should have a particular chemotherapy or radiation program, or ask too carefully what are the side effects and the likelihood of its being effective and then say that you want to think about the matter a bit, why, then you are obviously disturbed and neurotic and the department of psychiatry is called in to "adjust" you.

This viewpoint is much more prevalent in some places than

it is in others.* The obvious thing to do when a psychiatrist
visits you under these circumstances is to say politely "I did not
request your visit. I will not talk to you. I will refuse any bill you
send me. Please go away." Most psychiatrists will get the message. If they are too persistent, telephone the hospital administrator and say that there is an unauthorized person in your room
who refuses to leave. That should do the trick.

There are, however, many situations in which you may find
a hospital psychiatrist or psychologist very useful. If you feel that
your anxieties are overwhelming your ability to think clearly and
make good decisions, if you are troubled by strong depressive
feelings, if you cannot see any future for yourself, if you do not
know what to do next, then there may be a hospital psychiatrist
who is a mature human being with a well-trained and experienced mind with whom it can be very helpful to talk. Do not
be afraid or ashamed to ask for a psychiatric consultation. No
one will think you are crazy and it can be a very constructive
discussion. In situations where you need someone to discuss
serious matters with and the psychiatrist turns out to be too
young, inexperienced, or stupid, then in a surprisingly large
number of hospitals you will find the characteristics for which
you are looking in members of the chaplain's department.

Sometimes if you ask too many questions and appear to
doubt that all decisions of the medical staff are sent by God's
wisdom and absolutely correct, the physician will prescribe tranquilizers. These are to knock out your critical faculties and make
you more pliable; they thereby help you to become a good
patient who will not make anyone uncomfortable. Here is one
great advantage of having a strong advocate. No one can prescribe anything to zonk out *his or her* brain. You or your advocate *must* ask what is the name and purpose of every medication
prescribed (as well as what it looks like and when it will be
administered) and then you decide whether or not you want it.
Ask what it is supposed to do, what its side effects are, how

*The Psychiatry Department of New York City's famed Memorial Sloan-Ketter-
ing Cancer Center is particularly noted for this kind of activity.

effective it is. Then you decide. In many situations a tranquilizer may be very helpful. A severe illness can be a terrifying experience and often other terrors from our past combine to make it much more difficult for us to function. By all means take tranquilizers in this situation or in others when they are indicated. But you should remain in control of what agents you take to affect your brain. By and large, the more you are and stay in control of your own destiny, the better you will do. This approach may weaken the hospital staff's sense of omnipotence, but before you allow people to play God with you, make sure they have the qualifications!

Above all, don't be afraid to be difficult when something is wrong. If the sheets are not changed or your medication is not delivered reasonably on time, push your nurse's bell and complain. If you are bleeding and no one answers your bell—scream. In short, if you are in the hospital for the convenience of the staff, be a good patient. If you are there because you are sick and want to get the maximum benefits from your stay, then do everything possible to retain your adult status and as much control as you can over your own destiny.

If you have pain while in the hospital, do not be heroic about it. Every study shows that people who receive their pain medication when the pain first starts need much less of it and ask for it less often than do people who wait until they can't stand it anymore. The longer you wait, the more muscles in the area are going to tighten up and the more the pain will increase. The more sore and painful the whole area becomes because of muscle spasms, the less effect the pain medication will have and the more likely it is that the pain will quickly return after the medication wears off. Heroism is out of place in hospitals.

If you are not in a hospital but have to go to a hospital emergency room, having someone with you is also helpful. If the person can be a strong advocate who will stay until a decision has been made as to what the problem is and what to do about it, so much the better.

Let us say that it is 3:00 A.M. and you go to the emergency room with severe pain. If there is no one who can accompany you, while you are waiting for the ambulance, try to phone someone to meet you at the hospital. When you arrive, you or your advocate should make a fuss. Tell whoever is in charge loudly and clearly how severe your pain is and that you think you are going to faint. While the meek may inherit the earth, unless you are in a hurry to inherit your six feet of it, do not be meek. If the nurses or other staff say they are too busy to treat you immediately, or if the examining physician does not show up in a reasonable time, pick up a phone and call the administrative director. There is always one on duty. Or better, have your advocate go to his or her office and make a fuss there.

When you see the examining physician, you or your advocate should get his or her name. (Physicians, like other people, work better if someone is watching and knows who they are.) In addition, you or your advocate should ascertain (either then or, in some cases, in the morning) what examinations were made and what the diagnosis was.

In the emergency room follow the same general rules that apply to any hospital stay. Allow no arduous procedure until you understand why it is necessary and what the alternatives are. Be stubborn about this. It is likely to save you discomfort and money; it may save your life.

One last word about emergency rooms. Leave jewelry at home and bring only enough money to pay the required fees. Things have a habit of disappearing there.

In the past few pages, I have been discussing the negative aspects of many modern hospitals and have presented a very unfair and biased picture. I have emphasized these aspects in order to help people protect themselves. A more complete picture would take into account the fact that the modern hospital is far superior to any institution we have had in the past. Hospitals save a vast number of lives and prevent a vast amount of pain. One need only be very ill, or have an ill child, to experience the positive aspects as well. It is entirely legitimate to criticize the modern hospital system strongly so as to try to make it better and to help patients function better within it. It is also more legitimate to thank God that the modern hospital is there when we need it.

5

THE PROBLEM OF DESPAIR

"It's as if all my life I've been climbing a very steep mountain. It's very hard work. Every now and then there are ledges I can rest on and even enjoy myself for a little while. But I've got to keep climbing and the mountain I'm on has no top."

"I found I hated working for the union. It was too late to go back to music although I tried. I knew I'd have to stay in the business end for good. There was no way out, no matter what I did."

"The more I tried to tear it down, the higher and thicker became the wall of thorns I had built around myself. I couldn't get past it to other people. I feel like Dornrosen [the fairy-tale princess who slept inside a circle of thorns until a prince breached it and awakened her], except that the forest has grown so thick that no one will find me. The path is too overgrown ever to be used again."

"No matter what I did it didn't work. I lost my ability [to write] and so did Tom, and the more we tried, the worse it got. I gave up everything for him and—I see now—it destroyed us both. We had a mutual strangulation society. There just didn't seem any way out. . . . I often thought I'd only escape by dying."

"I'm like 'Rappaccini's Daughter' [a story by Hawthorne]. I need love and can respond to love, but I poison them [anyone she loves] because they don't have my immunity to my own poison. . . . I don't guess you or anybody else knows what it means to have no hope at all."

I have termed the orientation that these people seemed to be expressing "despair." A group of scientists led by William Greene and Arthur Schmale have called it "hopelessness." It is a deep and profound orientation that nothing you can do, or nothing that happens from the outside, can ever bring any real meaning and zest and enthusiasm to life.

One highly experienced internist who made a practice of carefully listening to his patients put it: "Patients with cancer, I believe, die from a negative state of stress so to speak. They die when they are overcome by a state of futility and hopelessness."

Mary had an intense drive, since childhood, to write poetry. Her view of herself and her reaction to the environment were in this frame of reference. Her work was of very high quality and could easily have been published, but she never was able to show it to anyone or to send it to a publisher, as she felt it would reveal how different she was from everyone else and would cause her to be rejected by others. After several months of therapy she—with much anxiety—showed some of her verse to the therapist who privately obtained a professional opinion of it. This corroborated his own impression that it was of very high caliber indeed, of close to first rank.

Mary had married a writer and—for a brief time—the relationship had been loving, mutually supportive, and intense. He was beginning his career and felt confident of his future development. When it became apparent that *her* abilities were far greater than his, her writing became a real threat to him, and he withdrew emotionally from their relationship. With her acute artistic perception Mary realized that her early anxieties—about whether to be a poet *or* be loved—now seemed justified by reality. She tried to give up her poetry, tried very hard to give up all of herself for him. The relationship, however, did not improve and presently she found herself unable either to write or to be loved, and was deeply despairing of any real satisfaction in her life.

In the early 1940s when I was beginning to learn about psychology, it was conventional wisdom in the field that each type of physical syndrome was associated with a particular type of personality pattern. Stomach ulcers were found in people with a large amount of repressed dependency needs, people with arthritis had a lot of repressed hostility, and so forth. Psychiatrists and psychologists of the very high caliber of Flanders Dunbar and Franz Alexander had done extensive and serious research leading to this viewpoint.

We have come a good distance since those days. Today we realize that when large groups of people are studied sometimes such relationships are found, but we recognize that no predictions from this kind of research can be made to individuals. The statistical tendencies often exist, but every person is unique and can be understood only in the context of his or her particular genetic endowment and life experience, and how they have interacted. Everyone is different and no one is cut exactly to a standard. With each of us, the day we were born, they broke the mold. We recognize now that if you know someone whose physical condition matches exactly the psychological pattern described in the textbooks, this means that you do not know the person very well.

One of the greatest errors in modern-day psychology and psychiatry has been the belief that the more we know, the more we will be able to use categories and mathematical formulas to describe and understand; that being able to put individual human beings into categories and assigning numerical values to them is a mark of our knowing a great deal about them. The reverse is actually true. Categorizing the person as a "this" or a "that" (for example, in the jargon of the third edition of the *Diagnostic and Statistical Manual of Mental Disorders*, diagnosing a person as a 309.28 or a 309.29) shows that we know very little about him. We know so little about the patient that we can describe him or her only in terms that also fit many thousands of others.

The error is rampant in psychology and psychiatry, but not limited to these fields. Bertrand Russell wrote in this context: "Physics is mathematical not because we know so much about the physical world, but because we know so little: it is only its mathematical properties that we can discover."

We know today that unless you can see, in someone with whom you are working, a full novel by Dostoevsky or a complete Shakespearean tragedy, you have only a superficial knowledge about the person. Each of us—I have seen no exceptions—lives in a full rich universe of our own, a universe full of pain, joy, hope, fear, sadness, regret, pride, loneliness, relationships, solitude, hates, loves, and everything else that artists and writers have shown us is part of the human condition. Even when we know someone else well, we still miss much of the intense color and flavor of their life. The philosopher and poet Goethe put it: "Gray are all your theories, but green the golden tree of life."

The universe of each of us is unique, duplicated by none other. Generalizations about human beings always limp; they are already inadequate when they are made. And yet they are useful tools. Like other types of concepts, they enable us to see and grasp what we would often otherwise miss. Just as the Impressionist artists such as Monet, Cézanne, Van Gogh, and Derain helped us to see the world in new ways—and thus helped greatly to bring into existence much of the modern scientific revolution—so does a concept help us see more possibilities than existed before for us. As tools, concepts can be used well or poorly. Without them we are limited. If, as the psychologist Abe Maslow once said, you only have a hammer, you must treat everything as a nail. But with other tools in your tool box or your mental armamentarium—your *apperceptive mass* in the older language—you can perceive and treat things and people with far more discrimination. It is for this reason that we find concepts of such value and that I introduce here the concept of *despair*.

Despair is the basic life orientation that emerged in most of the cancer patients during psychotherapy. Its verbalization often came as a surprise to the patients, followed swiftly by a realization that "this is how I always felt." All the evidence from long-term individual psychotherapy with these people indicated that the emotional orientation of despair predated the appearance of the cancer by many years. It had been the person's basic life-feeling, their *Lebensgefühl* for most of their lives. There had been periods in each life when this background music was very loud and periods when it was quite low, but it had always been there.

Once this feeling had emerged into consciousness, patients were often badly "flooded" by it for a long time. It kept reappearing in many forms and on many subjects until it could be finally worked through. This was an extremely painful time for the patients. However, once a more realistic orientation had replaced it, intelligent and constructive movement was possible in the patients' personalities and life space.

As the quotations given at the beginning of this chapter demonstrate, the patients related their despair only superficially to their cancer. Their fatal disease—all the patients studied knew their diagnosis and its usual prognosis—was seen as only "one more example" of the hopelessness of life for them. They felt that the despair long antedated the neoplasms and that their becoming fatally ill merely confirmed what they already believed. The problem of their unbearable existence was being solved for them by the cancer in a final, irrevocable getting rid of themselves. This was literally the solution they had always figuratively feared and yet felt was inescapable.

———————— ■ ————————

Nearly all of the people with cancer with whom I worked in the first fifteen years of this research had little hope from medical treatment. Either the accepted treatments had already failed, or experience had shown that there was little chance of saving these people's lives. Thus this was a special group within the cancer population, and it may be that the concept I am going to describe is applicable chiefly to this special population. I have seen it also in some recovering cancer patients and in a few people who did not have cancer at all. However, it was found in nearly all those cancer patients whom modern medicine could not help. It is more typical of this group than of any other I know. The fact that the only place I have seen it described elsewhere was in a book by Kierkegaard called *The Sickness Unto Death* is, perhaps, not a coincidence.

People in despair very often feel that there are only two roads open to them in life. They can be themselves, be, relate, create in their own way. If they do this, they will be alone as they view "their way" as a way of being that is not acceptable to others. The loneliness will be too great to bear. Or they can take the second path: they can adapt to the wishes and demands of others, they can bury their own uniqueness, their own individuality, and then they will be accepted by others and—in the words of one patient—"be given enough crumbs of love to almost survive." However, if they do take this second path, they will still feel basically alone. They are accepted by others for what they do, not what they are. Further, they will have joined the rest of the world in rejecting themselves, and this will be an additionally cruel and hard burden. With only these two paths perceived as possible, the outlook seems bleak indeed and the despair justified. One patient told me that all her life she had a slogan that seemed to sum up all the possibilities available to her. "If the rock drops on the egg—poor egg. If the egg drops on the rock—poor egg." It was clear to both of us that she identified herself with the egg, not with the rock. Whatever she did or whatever happened, the results would be the same—poor egg.

One patient saw it as a conflict between her "individuality" and "popularity"—to be herself or to be loved. "And it's as if I have to have both food and water to live and I can only have one of them." To give up her "individuality," her own way of seeing and reaching to the world, meant the loss of herself; to retain it meant being alone.

Early in therapy, this patient (a brilliant, highly trained specialist in her field) had expressed a great deal of anxiety about being a "mediocrity," an everyday type of person with no special features who could fit quite easily into her local suburban group. Exploration revealed that she knew she was unusual, but that she was afraid of her own drives deliberately to become a "mediocrity," to give up her special differences in order to try to win love and acceptance. Although she had much anxiety that she would do this, this particular patient was never able to accept the Faustian bargain: she could not sell her soul (as she saw the price demanded) for love, nor could she live without the water of love. Seeing only these two possible alternatives, she was filled with a deep despair about ever having a life worth living.

Another patient, in his first session, told how he had always been an independent person who "never needed a pillow" in his life. The qualities of strength, competence, dominance, and independence marked the central parts, the bone structure of his individuality, as he saw himself. This is what he was and had been. As the therapy progressed, however, it developed that he felt he could not be loved as himself, could only win fear and respect, and that to gain the love he so desperately needed he must become passive, dependent, and weak. He could not do this, and yet he felt he could not gain what he needed without doing it. Expending more and more energy in a frenzied attempt to gain love through domination and control, an attempt he

knew must fail and yet, as he saw no alternative, felt compelled
to continue, he deeply wished to die and thus be able to cease
the struggle.

People who are not in despair always have a hope that the
situation can be changed: perhaps by their own efforts, perhaps
by what happens accidentally around them (by actions and
occurrences outside themselves), or perhaps just by the very
passage of time itself. People in despair have lost all faith in these
possibilities: in the ability of their own actions, of outside
"objects" or occurrences, or of time to solve the problem. The
"mountain" they must climb has no top, and there is no way
for them to end the necessity of endless climbing.

They feel that no matter what they do, no matter how hard
or deviously they twist and turn to avoid their fate, it would
inexorably come. Any escapes were at best temporary, mere
"ledges [on the mountain] I can rest on . . ." and to believe in
their reality or permanence would only lead to a bitter disappointment.

One woman told me that since she was a child she had been
haunted by a story. She was not sure if it was a novel she had
read, a movie she had seen, or something she had made up
herself. But she remembered knowing it and visualizing it as
clearly as if she had been there, from as far back as she could
remember. In the story several people were fleeing in a car from
several cars full of murderous enemies following them. If they
could get over a long and difficult pass in the mountains, they
would be safe.

She visualized it as a movie. On the screen, the action of
the attempted escape and pursuit was interrupted from time to
time to show a large, dilapidated truck carrying a load of urinals
crossing the desert on the other side of the mountains and
approaching them. Gradually those fleeing for their lives drew
farther ahead of their pursuers. They began to believe they
would escape, and finally drove over the peak of the mountain
pass and started down the other side. At the same time, the
truckload of urinals began to climb the foothills. The outcome
was clearly foretold. Just as the protagonists became convinced

that they had successfully made their escape, they would be killed in a crash with the truck. "I always knew that, somehow, this was and would be the story of my life," she said.

The basic problem that underlies despair is the belief that the self cannot be accepted for what it is. If the self is seen as something that will be rejected by others, then the person is doomed to be eternally and deeply alone. If it is seen as something that one rejects oneself, the loneliness is made even greater. And if, as is often the case, the person feels both these conditions to be true, the life situation is as bleak and terrible as can be imagined. It is a hopeless bind. Kierkegaard, writing of the "disrelationship of despair," points out that to get rid of despair one must get rid of one's self, for it is one's self that one despairs of. But to get rid of one's self is also a cause of despair as it means to be no longer oneself, no longer to exist as the person you are. Over and over, in the people with cancer whom I saw, I found some formulation of this dilemma. Patients felt, clearly and consciously or at deeper personality levels, that to gain what they needed to bring meaning, zest, and enthusiasm to their lives they must give up themselves and become someone else. Even to consider this solution gave rise to despair, as they knew it would not and could not work. The love that they received for changing themselves into someone else was unacceptable to them; they were loved for what they did, not what they truly were, and this kind of love has very little nourishment in it.

In the twilight of his life, a year before he died, Freud was asked a profound question by one of his leading students. J. C. Flügel, the British psychoanalyst, asked him, "Tell me, Maestro, why does psychoanalysis *really* cure the patient?" Freud thought about it and then answered, out of his long experience and wisdom, "At one moment the analyst loves the patient and the patient knows it and the patient is cured."

As we look at this reply, it is clear why psychotherapy often takes so long. Patients must know that the analyst knows *who they truly are and loves them as they are.* Only when we are known for who we really are and loved for that can we *feel* loved and *accept* being loved.

Many of the people I worked with had, for one period or another, tried to deny what they saw as their true selves. It never succeeded in bringing them what they needed so desperately—the known love that would water and nourish their souls.

Once people face the fact that they are in despair, and that this has been part of the color of their life (Kierkegaard put it:· "Once a person is in despair, this shows that he has been in despair his whole life"), the question arises of how to solve the basic problem. Seeing the truth is often very hard and takes much time. The truth is that *the solution comes from becoming more and more the self you truly are.* The more this becomes your path and goal, then the more those who approve of the person you really are can recognize you and move toward you. By and large, these will be the kind of people *you* like, although there will be exceptions. Only after people in despair have had the courage to show their true face can these others recognize and respond with liking and love. And it is only after this—after finding and showing your true being—that love can be accepted and believed in.

This despair was so deep and hopeless in most of the people I saw that there was fairly little emotion connected with it. There was no rage or pain—it was part of their world and had always been as long as they remembered. "This is how I always felt," they would say. "This is how it always was with me." It was simply their environment.

> I tell you, hopeless grief is passionless;
>   That only men incredulous of despair
>   Half-taught in anguish, through the midnight air
> Beat upward to God's throne in loud access
> of Shrieking and Reproach. Full desertness,

In souls as countries, lieth silent-bare
Under the blanching, vertical eye-glare
of the absolute Heavens.
—ELIZABETH BARRETT BROWNING

Because it was so long and so basically a part of their picture of the world, their *Weltbild*, they had continued to function, gone on with the business of living, maintained the routine of their lives, and never believed that life could hold any real satisfaction or meaning for them. When we are depressed, we slow down; the deeper our depression, the less we do. In despair, however, we continue; we do not even have enough hope for meaning in life to be depressed about not being able to achieve it! Instead of slowing down and doing less, we continue with the hopeless grind of our lives.

Usually, in the people I saw, the despair was so deep and so much a part of them that even the appearance of the cancer and its diagnosis did not make a difference in how they maintained their daily lives. Even in the face of an out-of-control disease, they tended not to seek new experiences or to change their usual patterns of behavior. The cancer was not seen as something *new* in their lives, only as the latest and final example of the basic hopelessness that had so long been a part of their existence.

Occasionally, however, this was not true. And in these exceptions, there appeared to be a strengthening of the action of the person's cancer-defense mechanism. At the end of Chapter 2 (pp. 64–65), I recounted the story of Dr. Meerloo's patient who loved being on the sea. She was perhaps one example of this. Karen may be another.

Karen had been raised in a family in which there was a very great stress on the fact that a "good" person takes care of other people and puts his or her own needs second. Karen had always loved to draw. More than anything else, she wanted to be a commercial artist. Her family, however, did not view this as an occupation that contributed to the good of humanity, and it was therefore unacceptable. Karen therefore studied school administration in college and went into this field. As she put it, "Art is everything for me so I gave it up to take care of others. To do what I should." When I questioned her further on this, she said: "I was always taught that I must do the things I *should* do rather than what I want to do."

She was successful in her chosen career and rose fairly rapidly in the school system. She brought high intelligence and a high energy level to her work, and is one of those people who probably would have been successful in anything to which she applied herself, no matter what her personal likes and dislikes were about the field.

In her early thirties, she developed a rapidly growing breast cancer with metastases to the lymph nodes. She brought a large briefcase of papers from her office and planned to take care of them in the hospital while recuperating from a mastectomy.

The day before surgery was scheduled, Karen suddenly felt a great freedom. It was, she said, as if a tremendous load had been suddenly lifted from her shoulders. She felt, "I have cancer. Therefore I can now do what *I* want. I don't have to take care of these papers. I can *draw* again."

During her recuperation, she spent most of her time with a sketch pad and pencils instead of with the professional papers in her briefcase. The results of the mastectomy were excellent. No further symptoms were seen for seven years, after which a small node appeared on the scar tissue. A biopsy was inconclusive and further surgery was advised. Karen decided instead on a wait-and-watch policy. She started to pay even more attention to her needs as a person and as an artist. She took up working with watercolors, something she had wanted to do for a long time but "had just never gotten around to it." After three months, the node disappeared and no further symptoms were noted in the following ten years. She says her life is full and rich "and there is always so much more to learn how to do."*

In some of the other people I saw who had cancer, the despair seemed so deep and pervasive that nothing I could do could shake it and they were not able to overcome it themselves. One of these was Roslyn.

During her adolescence she had been deeply and profoundly idealistic. She felt for the hungry and the oppressed everywhere on Earth. She worked with organizations for good causes, was a volunteer in a settlement house in New York City, and finally decided that she could do the most good as a teacher of young children.

During her college years, she became aware of the great promise of peace, economic security, and hope offered by Marxism. She joined the Communist Party as they, it seemed to her, were the only ones both working actively for the hungry and homeless now and also offering them a program for the future.

In the Party, she was dedicated and active. With her great idealism, she never permitted her political beliefs to come into the classroom, where she felt that they did not belong, but after hours she worked long and hard at everything from passing out leaflets to lobbying for specific bills. Roslyn also attended several political meetings a week. At night, she said, "I can never go to sleep until I have read today's *New Masses* [the daily Communist newspaper of the period] and found out the truth about what is going on in the world." Too idealistic to

---

*Psychotherapists wishing for further analysis of this orientation of despair may be interested in an article of mine, "A Psychological Orientation Associated with Cancer," *The Psychiatric Quarterly*, no. 3 (1971): 141.

rise high in the Party ranks, she was one of its most faithful and hardworking members.

The Party formed the total context and center of her life. The future hope of the communist state gave meaning to everything she did. She and her husband, also a Party member, had wanted to have children, but they gave up the idea as they were so busy with Party work that they felt they did not have the time and energy needed to raise children properly and with the affection they would need. Knowing that they were frequently followed by government agents, that their telephone was often tapped, that there were many paths of vocational advancement closed to them—these were parts of their everyday life and of the suffering that they accepted in terms of future goals for the human race.

Roslyn's husband, a quiet, low-energy, serious high school principal, was blacklisted and lost his job during the McCarthy period. For many years thereafter he stayed at home and kept house while she supported them financially. She loved her work as a nursery school teacher and the little ones in her care.

In the early 1960s, it became possible for her to fulfill a lifelong dream and make her first visit to the USSR. Here, where communism had been in existence for over forty years, she would be able to see what the fruits of all her labor would look like in full bloom. Knowing that she would make the trip, she began two years in advance to study Russian. By the time she was ready to go, this highly intelligent and capable woman spoke the language fluently.

She spent six weeks in the Soviet Union, most of the time touring schools and kindergartens, as these were her major interest and area of greatest training. She was horrified at what she found. The rigidity with which the children were treated, the political brainwashing, the promotion of teachers and administrators on the basis of Party membership and orthodoxy rather than on ability and involvement with what was best for the children, the difference with which children were treated on the basis of their parents' social class; all these things could not be hidden from her trained and experienced eye. Both she and her husband were "sick at heart—we felt as if our lives and suffering were wasted" when they returned home.

She resigned from the Communist Party and gave up all her political activity. Her closest friends had all been Party members, and now none would speak to her. She continued teaching and her husband found an administrative job with a private school. "But the heart had gone out of our lives." I told her the phrase from Pericles' speech to the parents of the young men killed in battle: "It is as if the spring had gone out of the year." She said, "That's exactly how it feels to both of us."

Three months later she was diagnosed with a rapidly growing breast cancer that quickly spread to her lungs. She died within one year of her return from the Soviet Union.

6

THE HOLISTIC APPROACH TO HEALTH

. . . [Among the Greeks] eminent physicians say to a patient who comes to them with bad eyes, that they cannot cure his eyes by themselves, but that if his eyes are to be cured, his head must be treated; and then again they say that to think of curing his head alone, and not the rest of the body also, is the height of folly. And arguing in this way they apply these methods to the whole body, and try to treat and heal the whole and the part together. . . .

[The physicians from Thrace, however, criticize this and say that they are right as far as they go, but] that as you ought not to attempt to cure the eyes without the head, or the head without the eyes, neither ought to attempt to cure the body without the soul; and this . . . is the reason why the cure of so many diseases is unknown to the physicians of Hellas because they are ignorant of the whole, which ought to be studied also; for the part can never be well unless the whole is well.

PLATO, Charmides (Jowett translation)

Tom was a successful business executive in his mid-forties. He had joined his present company seventeen years before, with the presidency of the company as his goal. Now he had been prom-

116

ised that he would be promoted to this position within a year. The center of his world was his work at which, apparently, he was very good indeed. He had been married for fifteen years to a chic, intelligent, and ambitious career woman who worked in a field allied to his own. Both loved skiing and they took regular vacations in Switzerland and in Sun Valley. He described the marriage as "Okay, no problem," and she concurred with this opinion.

Two months before he was to move into the new job, a number of suddenly appearing symptoms brought him to his physician. A rapidly advancing Hodgkin's disease was diagnosed. (At this time Hodgkin's was considered an invariably fatal diagnosis by all serious medical opinion.)

At that time, as part of my research, I was routinely interviewing every fourth patient who came through the outpatient cancer service. During the first interview Tom told me that he felt his cancer "had something to do with, maybe was caused by, my emotions." (I had found that cancer patients often expressed this idea, if they felt their listener might be receptive, although it was then almost unknown in medical circles. I'm reminded of John Dewey's statement that the person who is wearing the shoe knows where it pinches.) I asked him if he wanted to start on a program to explore this idea. He did, and so we started on a psychotherapy program.

Among the first things that came up in the therapy was that he was specialist in (among other things) information retrieval. When he realized how much he had been relying on others' opinions and knowledge about his condition, he looked surprised. He went to a medical library and learned all he could about Hodgkin's disease. Not liking at all the results that mainline medicine was obtaining, he began to add other approaches to the radiation prescribed by his physician. An osteopath whom he consulted recommended that he continue the radiation and in addition prescribed a number of sessions of osteopathic manipulation. Tom reported that these made him feel a good deal better and that he seemed to have much more energy after them than he had had before.

Then he looked for a nutritionist. It was hard, at that time, to find one who had the required balance of common sense, training, and experience with catastrophic illness, but after some search, Tom managed to do so. He went on a strict vegetarian diet with heavy vitamin and mineral supplements. The diet was not one that would be recommended by many nutritionists today, but it was the best advice available at the time.

During the course of psychotherapy, it quickly became apparent to Tom that his marriage was a pretty empty shell. The couple *liked* each other and had worked out a "pleasant" modus vivendi. Both he and his wife had settled for something very far from ideal. There was really very little to hold them together except habit and the belief that both seemed to share that nothing better was possible. We began to explore Tom's deep hopelessness and despair about ever attaining any really meaningful relationships. At one point he said to me, "You know how it is, Doc, in a house with no insulation. No matter how much heat you put into it, you can't get warm. You can only do that by having some of the heat reflected back at you. I always knew that that's how it was with me in life. No matter how hard I tried, no matter how much heat I put out, I would never be able to get warm." Working through this despair, which stemmed from early childhood, was a long and painful task.

When he began to realize how little he had settled for emotionally and how much more was possible for him, he and his wife began, for the first time, to talk with each other about their marriage. They went to a marriage counselor together and had several sessions with him. Then, suddenly, the wife was offered an excellent promotion if she would relocate to San Francisco. This seemed to clinch it for both of them. They divorced in an amiable and friendly manner. Both appeared to be quite relieved by this solution.

For a time, after the divorce, Tom felt that he wanted no relationships other than those he found in his work. Of course, we discussed this in the psychotherapy sessions. The fear behind it was explored and worked through. Presently he began to date and saw a number of women a few times each. After about a year, one of these relationships developed into an affair and then into marriage. The second wife is much more warm, open, and loving than the first had been. At one time I reminded Tom of his comments about the house with no insulation. He thought about it for a few moments, grinned, and said, "I feel much warmer now."

In psychotherapy we also explored at some length Tom's work. He realized that the job at which he had been aiming all these years seemed to him to be a dead end. What he really enjoyed was the challenge and the stimulation of new problems to be solved in new and ingenious ways. Once he had been through the cycle of problems that a new job presented a couple of times, he was bored at what seemed to him to be more routine. A new job was fascinating at first and then became a boring routine that he was doing while he waited to move on. Once he became president of the company, there would be no place to move on to. He would be, he felt, "all dressed up and no place to go. Ever!"

Further, he was aware that even the promise of the top job in his industry, with its implied recognition, had not really satisfied him. He saw that he was missing something in his life and that he had always known this and had, without being too conscious of doing this, counted on the "right" job, the biggest promotion, to solve his inner feelings of discontent with himself. When we talked about the fact that inner problems must be solved in their own sphere, that whatever happens in the outside world does not solve them, he quoted from the song "Adelaide's Lament" in Frank Loesser's musical comedy *Guys and Dolls*. In this, Adelaide tells how she develops a cold each time her marriage is put off, and that she could take all the patent medicines "but the medicine never gets anywhere near where the trouble is." We agreed that this was very true for him.

When Tom began to understand his feelings about his job's being a dead end, he also began to see the fallacy of the fantasy. The board had promised him this job because of his ability to make innovative decisions. They *wanted* him to take the company in new directions, and his brief was an open-ended one.

His employers clearly hoped he would continue to be creative and would develop the company in new ways. With this realization, Tom's despair over his work began to disappear.

The similar quality of the hopelessness he had felt over both his vocational and his emotional life and the sudden appearance of a catastrophic disease reminded me of Jung's statement: "When an inner situation is not made conscious, it appears outside as fate." Tom thought about this for a few long moments and then nodded in complete and very sad agreement.

I kept pointing out to him that he was doing beautifully in the spheres of existence directly relating to the psychotherapeutic process, but there were two others he had not been concerned with—the physical and the spiritual. If he wanted his treatment to be a holistic health approach, he had to work in these areas also. In the physical realm, the nutrition and the mainline medicine were part of it, but more was needed. He also needed a program of physical activity of a kind that was right for *him* now, at this stage of his development. Checking each time with his oncologist, he experimented with a number of forms of such activity. He joined a athletic club in which there were a large number of activities ranging from yoga to judo. He tried a number in an attempt to find one that felt right to him and would help with the necessary upgrading of his physical being. Finally he found that swimming laps in the pool was exactly what he wanted. He would go to the club in the early mornings when the pool was empty and slowly swim dozens of laps with his mind focused only on the swimming. He would generally emerge from the pool feeling slightly "high," "well put together," calm and energetic.

Understanding (intellectually only at this point) that he was not expressing or nourishing the spiritual part of his nature, and that was for him a real lack, Tom began to try to experiment with and to discover this part of himself. He knew from our discussions that the spiritual part of us needs to be nourished in two ways. First, and possibly least important for Westerners, is in one of the hard disciplines of meditation or prayer. Second, in active work that shows our concern for more than ourselves and our immediate families—for others, our species, or our planet.

The meditation program he settled on was an Eastern breath-counting exercise. Tom started doing this regularly for half an hour a day. On days he meditated, he found he felt more energetic and less "flappable" all day, more at home with himself and with others.

About a year after he began meditating, a client came into town who was going, one evening, to a meeting of the American Association for the United Nations. Tom attended with him, became interested, and is now a senior officer of the local chapter and is active on several national committees.

Tom's Hodgkin's disease responded well to the radiation program and the tumors regressed. They did not appear again for six months. At that time another course of radiation was given and they again disappeared. They have not, in the over twenty years since then, reappeared. In this time, Tom has changed his diet, his exercise, and his meditation program several times. What is right for us at one stage of our development is not in others. He worked at the post he was promoted to for about eight years and then moved to another company at a higher salary. He enjoys his work. His marriage is a good one and he has two children. Tom rates his life as "diverse, exciting and fascinating. The only problem is that there are only twenty-four hours in each day and I have about thirty-six hours of things I like to do."

Tom's way of dealing with his illness illustrates a new approach to health and disease that has appeared on the medical scene in the past twenty years. It is growing very rapidly and having an increasingly major effect on medical concepts and techniques. It is usually called *holistic medicine* or *holistic health*. In order to understand and use this approach, it is necessary to first look at a little of its history.

Ever since classical Greek times, there have been two basic viewpoints in Western medicine. The first (the "allopathic" view) has held that the physician should be someone who works actively against disease and illness, who strongly intervenes with whatever tools available—surgery, chemicals, and so on. The second (the "naturopathic" view) has held, rather, that the physician be someone who cooperates with the natural healing powers of the body and, by strengthening and supporting these, helps the patient to grow toward health.

Neither viewpoint has ever gone to complete extremes (except in the case of a few kooky groups). Even those with the most extreme naturopathic views have always recognized that if you had an artery cut and spouting blood, this was no time to discuss life-styles, nutrition, or spiritual practices—what you needed was someone who would actively intervene with a needle and thread! Similarly the most extreme devotees of surgery and chemicals have always known that the surgeon cannot heal the surgical wound; all he or she could do is to place the edges as carefully together as possible, keep the wound as clean as possible, and let the natural self-repair abilities of the patient do the healing.

In spite of this, however, there have been real differences of emphasis at different periods and in different places, and this has led to great difference in medical methods.

In Roman times, the conflict between those who believed in the healing powers of the body and in cooperating with them (the Hippocratics) and those who believed that this passive approach was useless, a mere "meditation on death," and that active intervention was necessary (the followers of Asclepiades of Bithynia) became even greater than it had been before. There was violent argument and vituperation on both sides.

The idea of the importance of the body's restorative and self-healing powers was not lost after the classical period, but was typical of the medieval approach. Thus according to the theory of humors (the accepted medical theory of the period), it was

believed that illness was due to an excess of one of the four kinds
of fluid in the body and that, when this condition occurred,
certain self-healing dispositions of the body automatically went
into action. For example, these dispositions raised the body
temperature so as to "cook" the excess of raw fluid and then
separate the cooked from the uncooked parts. Physicians *cooper-
ated* with these self-restorative dispositions. They gave warming
drinks and warmed the patient externally to help with the cook-
ing. They then helped the body to dispose of the cooked excess
by giving purges and emetics and by bleeding. Thus from the
medieval viewpoint, every disease was a process that physicians
could help regulate by cooperating with the patient's self-healing
abilities.

With the end of the medieval period however, a gradual
shift in viewpoint took place. By the beginning of the eighteenth
century, medical opinion throughout Europe and America was
primarily on the side of active intervention. Physicians saw their
task as that of taking arms against the disease process. However,
their knowledge and tools were as scant and ineffective as ever;
neither they nor those who espoused the "natural" healing
methods were able to do much good. Neither school knew very
much and, what was worse, most of what they were sure they
knew was wrong. Both killed people by the hundreds of thousands. The "naturopaths" probably obeyed to a much greater
degree Hippocrates' "first law" (*"Primum non nocere"*: "Above
all, do no harm") because they acted less aggressively and their
remedies were weaker. This may be the reason that in the early
1800s public opinion began to favor their approach.

On one side was the Popular Health Movement (PHM) and
on the other the orthodox physicians. The PHM used mostly
plant and herbal remedies and attacked the mainline physicians
for their "barbaric" treatments, fees, and "arrogance." They
sought to "return medicine to the people," to "make every man
his own doctor." Politically they worked through "Samuel
Thompson's Friendly Botanical Societies." Opposing them were
many leading physicians, such as the French F. J. U. Broussais,
who believed only active measures could cure disease since the

body had no natural healing power. In the event, the PHM and its allies were so successful that in the United States, state after state repealed its laws licensing physicians, and by 1849 only New Jersey and the District of Columbia had such laws still on the books. Elsewhere anyone was at liberty to hang up a shingle and go into practice as a physician. Mainline medicine, now known as "allopathic" medicine, seemed in complete rout and retreat.

It was at this time, however, that medicine made the two greatest advances in its history: the germ theory and the alliance with chemistry. Out of these came not only antiseptic and painless surgery, but one after the other of the great killer diseases were brought under control. Cholera, black plague, yellow fever—these and other diseases had ravaged the human race since its beginning, destroying civilizations and changing the course of history again and again. Now they were no longer to be feared. With this triumph, the pendulum swung again to the opposite extreme and mainline medicine took on an authority and prestige greater than at any previous time. Naturopathic medicine became considered the province of charlatans and primitives. The body's self-healing abilities were largely forgotten.

The extreme mechanistic approach that mainline medicine developed worked well for the great communicable killer diseases. But it did not work at all well for the degenerative diseases such as cancer, lupus, or various heart conditions. Largely for this reason, in recent years a new viewpoint has been appearing. This concept, holistic medicine, is, for the first time in our history, an *integration* of the two approaches, taking the best from each and using them in conjunction to potentiate each other.

Holistic medicine is a series of concepts, not a series of techniques. It rests on four basic axioms, four ideas that together form a coherent whole.

1. The person exists on many levels, all of which are equally real and important. Physical, psychological, and spiritual levels are one valid way of describing the person, and none of these can be "reduced" to any other. To move successfully toward health, all must be treated. All must be taken care of and gardened if health is to be maintained.

2. Each person is unique. A valid program of treatment, whether it focuses primarily on nutrition, meditation, chemotherapy, or exercise, must be individualized for each person. A standardized approach to a condition is not valid under this concept.

3. The patient should be a part of the decision-making team. Each person in a program of holistic health is given as much knowledge and authority as he or she will accept.

4. The person has self-healing abilities. Following the first three axioms helps to mobilize these abilities and bring them to the aid of the mainline medical program.*

Looking back at Tom, we can see how these four axioms were followed. His work toward health was on physical, psychological, and spiritual levels. Work on each level was highly individualized for him—he made the major decision after getting as much information as he could. His self-healing abilities were mobilized and came to the aid of the radiation program.

Let's examine these four axioms in a little more detail.

A person exists on many levels. The spiritual level cannot be reduced to or explained in terms of the psychological, nor can the psychological be explained in terms of the physical. Each is equally valid and must be dealt with in its own terms. On the physical level we have nutrition, medicine and surgery, exercise and movement programs. On the psychological level we deal with and try to upgrade in their functioning the kind of areas of the person that the psychotherapist deals with in his or her

*I have discussed the history and the concept of holistic health and the four axioms it rests on in detail in my book *The Mechanic and the Gardener: How to Understand and Use the Holistic Revolution in Medicine* (New York: Holt, Rinehart & Winston, 1982).

work: feelings and reactions to the self, others, and to that general nature of which we are all a part.

The hardest level to define has been the "spiritual." This word means so many things to so many people that there is vast confusion about it. In order to be able to work in this field effectively, we have had to define the term to include the two kinds of action, meditative and in-the-world. The first, the meditative, consists of one of those rigorous and disciplined practices of prayer or meditation that leads the person to the knowledge that he or she is a part of the total universe and cannot be meaningfully separated from it; to the full comprehension that his or her feelings of loneliness, alienation from others, and separateness are, in part, illusion. Whether one calls this "cosmic consciousness," "satori," "Christ consciousness," or what have you does not matter very much. This is an approach to, a feeding of, a part of the self that has been recognized and taught in every culture of which we know.

The second aspect relates particularly to Westerners, since in the West emphasis in spiritual growth has always been more on what you did than on how you felt. We are concerned with action. I do not regard a patient as finished until he or she is spending some time and energy in work demonstrating concern for more of the human race than the self and immediate family. I have former patients working in the Big Brothers, Big Sisters, ecology and peace organizations, in the Fortune Society, and many other similar areas. St. John of the Cross wrote: "If you were in an ecstasy as deep as that of St. Paul, and a sick man needed a cup of soup, it were better for you that you returned from that ecstasy and brought him the soup for love's sake." In the West we have always been clear about our priorities in spiritual development.

One very important thing needs to be added here. There are a large number of people with cancer who have spent a great deal of their time and energy taking care of others and very little taking care of themselves. This is *not* what we are talking about here. Before one protects and gardens others, one must learn to do this for the self. Timing is crucial here.

It is essential that the person first learns to sing their own song fully and then, as part of their human needs, finds a way to express their spiritual concern with others or with the human race as a whole. Only in this way do we act and live as a coherent whole and only in this way can we strengthen and mobilize our self-healing and self-repair abilities. If we are first for ourselves and are beating out our own music in being, relating, creating, then we also find that we are concerned with others, not as a replacement for caring for ourselves but out of selfish motives. The need to express our own spiritual needs has been part of the human being in every culture of which we have any records. It has been expressed all through human history, when people have sacrificed physical well-being for spiritual fulfillment. We know that the spiritual is a real part of us. When we have cancer and need to bring *all* of us to bear in our work toward health, we cannot afford to ignore any of our levels. They are too basic a part of being human not to cultivate if we wish to help our immune systems function.

The second axiom of holistic medicine is that each person is unique and each program must be individualized. Just as there is no one general right length of a therapy session or one right relationship between patient and psychotherapist, there is no one right diet or right exercise program or right amount and pattern of administration of medication that applies to everyone diagnosed with a particular condition. Each person must be treated as an individual and must determine, in large part by his or her own reactions, what is the best approach and process for him or her. As Francis Bacon put it: "There is a wisdom in this beyond the rules of physic [medicine]: A man's own observations, what he finds good of, and what he finds hurt of, is the best physic to preserve health."

The great teachers of spiritual development in the West have always understood that in psychic and spiritual development, there is a different path for each person.*

---

*The founder of modern Chassidic mysticism, the Ba'al Shem Tov, put it this way: "Every man should know that since creation no other man was ever like him. . . . Each is called on to perfect his unique qualities."

In her autobiography, St. Thérèse of Lisieux wrote of the problems of being a spiritual director:

> I know it seems easy to help souls, to make them love God above all, and to mold them according to His will. But actually, without His help it is easier to make the sun shine at night. One must banish one's own special tastes and personal ideas and guide souls along the special way Jesus indicates for them rather than along one's own particular way.

When the Seer of Lublin was asked to name one general way to the service of God, he replied:

> It is impossible to tell men the way they should take. For one way to serve God is through learning, another through prayer, another through fasting, and still another through eating. Everyone should carefully observe what way his heart draws him to, and then choose this way with all his strength.

In a similar vein, Rabbi Nachman of Bratislava wrote: "God calls one man with a shout, one with a song, one with a whisper."

In a similar vein, Rabbi Nachman of Bratislava wrote: "God calls one man with a shout, one with a song, one with a whisper." And spiritual leaders such as St. Theresa of Avila and Thomas Merton have pointed out that the path of inner development is different for each person, that each must work on his or her development in an individual way.

It is hard to overemphasize the importance of this point. So accustomed are we to believing that there is one right way to do things that doctors tend automatically to slip into treating patients according to this concept. The belief is strengthened by long years of medical education that emphasizes one cause for each disease and one correct procedure to follow in combating it.

Yet we differ tremendously from each other in our genetic heritage, in our childhood and adult experience of the world, in the degree and ways that we have nurtured or repressed our different needs, in the amount and ways we have directed our energies inward and outward, in our fears of ourselves and others, and in the meaning we have found for our lives. Knowledge of these differences is not just of theoretical interest but is crucial for work at all levels of the treatment of disease and the search for health. One reason a trained anesthesiologist is required at every major surgical procedure is that each person differs in response to an anesthetic and unless we want the patient to either die on the table or wake up screaming in the middle of the surgery, we have to monitor and adjust the amount constantly during the entire operation. Mainline medicine learned this the hard way when it first started to use anesthetics. In spite of careful attempts to predict in advance what a patient of *this* age and *this* weight and *this* condition would need, many patients did wake up screaming under the knife or else died of overdoses. Unfortunately mainline medicine has been very slow in applying the lesson in other areas.

A responsible physician today will, however, apply this lesson to many medical situations. If a patient needs a tranquilizer, the physician will not choose one that is the most popular one in the general classification desired, but will hand-tailor the prescription to the particular patient and then will monitor its effect at frequent intervals. He or she knows that no two people respond to the same chemical intervention in the same way.

Sara, a woman in her late forties, had achieved a very high position in public relations. She disliked her work but felt that it was impossible to give up such success. Her marriage was, as she described it, "friendly," but there was little love or warmth in it. It was a routine relationship between two people who had learned to "accommodate" to each other, but that was about all. There were no children.

Abdominal symptoms brought her to a medical examination, at which a stomach cancer with metastases was diagnosed. A chemotherapy program was recommended, but with little optimism. The prognosis was seen as poor. Her husband was told to expect that she would have a fairly rapid decline and would probably die within eighteen months.

Her husband, who did respect his wife as an adult, listened

to her plea that she wanted *all* the truth, and told her exactly what the oncologist had told him. Sara then decided that the medical program as outlined did not hold enough promise to be worth undertaking, particularly as the side effects of the chemotherapy were likely to be very severe.

She determined to design her own program from whatever sources were available and began first to investigate alternative cancer treatments. She decided that since she did not have the training to evaluate the biochemical and cellular aspects of the various treatment programs, she would use her years of experience in business to evaluate the person in charge of each one. She met and talked with about a dozen physicians who were using alternative methods and chose the one who seemed to her to be of the highest personal caliber. (They all seemed to make about the same claims for success and personality was the only indicator that she felt competent to use.)

Sara regarded her medical treatment as the cornerstone of her approach to the cancer, but felt that it was far from sufficient. She began to investigate other domains of her being. She started with a nutrition program that made sense to her and that her physician assured her was not contraindicated by the medical treatment. (He also assured her that it was useless and would not do her any good, but she ignored his opinion as he had had absolutely no training in the field.) Investigating exercise and movement programs, she was unable to follow her first choice—folk dancing—because of her illness, but she found a great deal of enjoyment in a thrice-weekly sensory awareness (Gindler method) class. She began to feel more at home in her body and more related to it than she had ever felt before in her life. She began to study a form of meditation and meditated twice a day for twenty minutes each time. She started psychotherapy with a therapist whose orientation was on helping her patients find out what was "right" for them (in what ways of being, relating, and creating they would find the fullest joy, zest, and serenity) and what was blocking their expression, rather than on finding out what was "wrong" with them. As a result of the therapy, Sara decided that a large paycheck and a lot of prestige were not enough return for spending forty of her best hours each week at a job she hated. She resigned and started a new career (in personnel guidance), which she thoroughly enjoyed. Rather than dreading each new day, Sara found she was glad to get up every morning to go to the office. She was earning far less than before but was enjoying her life much more.

Two evenings a week, she works on a volunteer basis at the Fortune Society, a group devoted to helping former convicts turn their lives around. She teaches reading and coaches group members who are applying for office jobs or are starting them in how to behave in an office, how to dress, relate, and so on. She loves this work and says, "It feeds a part of me I never knew was there." Many others who have begun volunteer work for the first time say something similar.

As Sara began to grow and change, she insisted that her husband also change. After some badgering, he also started in psychotherapy. As they both grew emotionally, they discovered that they liked each other more. (Their relationship could, of course, have gone the other way and ended in divorce.) The marriage improved considerably and for the first time became alive and vital.

The year after Sara started the medical program, her tumors regressed. Six years later she is now symptom free, and X rays show no sign of cancer.

It is, of course, entirely possible that she would have responded to the medical treatment without the work on other levels. She even might have responded to the original chemotherapy program as outlined so pessimistically by her first oncologist. We simply cannot know. What she did, however, was to maximize her chances of responding positively. She approached the problem on as many levels of her being as possible and thereby made it much more likely that her self-healing abilities would be fully mobilized. She also improved the general quality of her life to a very considerable extent and certainly made it more worth living for whatever time she did have.

By taking her destiny into her own hands and designing a unique and individual multilevel program for herself, Sara had followed exactly what we would say today is the basic viewpoint of holistic medicine.

Sensory awareness, the adjunctive modality that Sara used in the body sphere, is a method of becoming *aware* of ourselves through physical sensations. In lying, sitting, standing, or during very slow movements, you try to become as conscious as possible of the sensations of the body. There is a deep total and gentle concentration on what is going on in the body and in the breathing. You begin to understand how much you have separated yourself from the body and the parts of the body from each other. You realize that the lack of attention to bodily sensations is an aspect of the fragmentation of the self and recognize how far this has progressed. You generally leave a session feeling far different (and much better) physically and emotionally than when entering. The instructor suggests what part of the body to focus the attention on. As you heal the splits within the self, the gulfs between the self and others and between the self and the general nature of which we are all a part tend to lessen. This Western form of *hatha* (physical) yoga was developed in the 1920s in Germany by Elsie Gindler.*

The form of meditation Sara used is widely used today. It involves the use of a *mantra,* a very old meditation method in which the individual, as physically relaxed as possible, repeats over and over to him- or herself a chosen phrase. Each time the mind wanders it is gently brought back to the repetition. The classical explanation for the effectiveness of this method is that the carefully chosen phrase has a positive effect on the individual it was chosen for. More modern theory suggests that it is the doing of just one thing at a time, involving as much of the being as possible in a deliberately chosen single activity, that has the desired effect. Thus some researchers have suggested that any simple (preferably meaningless) word or phrase will do.

In any case, if this meditation is done conscientiously twice a day for twenty minutes at a time, it certainly tends to have

*The best-known teachers of this method today are Charlotte Selver and Corolla Speads.

positive effects on the meditator. Greater feelings of calmness and ability to cope and a normalization of such variables as blood pressure and blood acid-alkalinity levels have been widely reported.

■

Abraham Meyerson, one of the great American psychiatrists, used to say in his classes: "As soon as you have decided on the basis of long experience and theory that all patients who have A also have B, and that this can be absolutely depended on, you can be completely certain that within three days, a patient will come into your office with A and not the slightest sign of B. This will happen. The only question is will you be too blind to see it." Unfortunately, a large percentage of health professionals of all kinds are chronically blind in this direction. They are so certain of their theories and experience that they are unable to notice individual differences. Such blindness kills a lot of people.

(Many of these professionals will defend themselves by saying, "I have had twenty years of experience in this field and . . ." What they really mean, of course, is "I have had one year of experience repeated twenty times and I have not learned anything in nineteen years!")

The third axiom is that the patient should be as much a part of the decision-making team as he will accept. One very knowledgeable physician, Marvin Meitus, from whom I have learned a great deal about holistic medicine, put it:

The patient must participate in his own treatment. He must help himself to get well. Participation is more than taking a pill every day. He must choose a diet, exercise, relaxation, and so forth. Pretty soon you get patients who are no longer taking pills . . . The miracle cure is when the patient helped cure himself . . . It's more important what you don't do for a patient than

what you do do . . . When a patient says, "What can I do to
help?" you are in a new ball game.

Patients are the world's outstanding authorities on how
they themselves feel. They know the ground of their life, its
color and texture better than anyone else. The health professional has a wider view and is more knowledgeable than patients
in many of the problems and therapies relating to health. Working together they can form an effective and smoothly functioning team, but only patients can judge how they feel, or whether
a particular procedure is helping or not. They are alone in the
midst of their life and experience it directly. Even gifted with the
greatest possible training and empathy, the health professional
is still at a distance.

A program to improve the self-care of patients with diabe-
tes at the University of Southern California resulted in a 50
percent reduction in emergency ward visits, a decrease in the
number of patients with diabetic coma from 300 to 100 over a
two-year period, and the avoidance of 2,300 visits for medication. Savings were estimated at $1.7 million.

A large number of similar studies and experiments have
demonstrated without question that medical results are far superior when patients have been made a member of the decision-
making team than when decisions about health and illness are
made autocratically by someone else. When patients are involved in the decisions, the results of the particular program
tend to be markedly better, there are fewer negative side effects,
and patients tend to sue less often!

The fourth axiom is that people have self-healing abilities.
Following the first three axioms helps to mobilize these and
bring them to the aid of the mainline medical program.

The importance of our self-healing abilities has, perhaps,
been shown nowhere more clearly than in work in recent years
on the *placebo effect.* This term has been found in medical
dictionaries since 1811. Patients who receive a placebo (a sub-
stance that will have no biological effect on the problem—sugar
of milk has often been used) often show remarkable positive

results if they and the administering physician both believe it is an important new treatment guaranteed to cure the condition. Medicine has generally regarded the placebo effect as a nuisance: it does make research on new medical drugs very difficult. Ignoring it has slowed medical progress considerably in two ways. First, the role of the patient's own attitudes and self-repair systems in recovery has been obscured. Second, many medications and surgical procedures have been used and have worked well until the physician's enthusiasm waned. Excellent reviews of this subject are given in Brian Inglis's *The Case for Unorthodox Medicine* and in Jerome Frank's *Persuasion and Healing.** The following paragraphs from Inglis's book may serve as an example.

> In the summer of 1962, a report was published of a test of three drugs used in the treatment of the agonizing paroxysmal pain known as angina pectoris: iproniazid, which had been thought to be highly effective, but had liver damage as occasional side effect; malamide, less toxic, but also presumed to be rather less effective; and the tranquilizer meprobamate, again. All three were tested double blind, with placebo controls, and more patients responded better to the placebo than to any of the drugs. The authors concluded that earlier enthusiastic reports of improvement based on uncontrolled trials were probably due "to temporary changes in the mental outlook of the individual patients concerned, or to natural variations in the symptoms."
>
> Such tests bred disillusionment; and it was not only over drugs; if placebo effect was so extensive, physicians countered, might it not be responsible for the "success" of many surgical operations? A great deal of evidence has accumulated to show that this has indeed been the case. In the 1920's, for example, it became fashionable to treat duodenal ulcers by gastroeneterostomy [sic]; such famous surgeons as W. J. Mayo in the United States and Lord Moynihan in Britain used it extensively. It seemed eminently sensible, since it formed a communication be-

*Jerome Frank, *Persuasion and Healing* (Baltimore: Johns Hopkins Press, 1961).

tween the stomach and the small intestine, bypassing the pylorus where ulcers originated, *"permitting of the discharge of gastric contents into the duodenum, where they belong,"* (as one enthusiast described it), *"and allowing the alkaline duodenal contents to pass back into the stomach for the neutralization of gastric acids."* Reports were at first almost uniformly gratifying: it was claimed that about 80 percent of patients operated on were still cured five years later, less than two percent suffering from ulcers elsewhere. But eventually a source hostile to the operation reported that the incidence of these *"marginal"* ulcers following the operation was far higher—in the region of 33 percent; the operation fell out of favor; and it has even been stated that any surgeon using it now would leave himself open to a suit for malpractice.

Since the 1920's, many other forms of treatment of stomach ulcers may have been temporarily fashionable; but there is good reason to believe that their successes, too, have been due to placebo effect. In his Persuasion and Healing, Dr. Jerome Frank of the Johns Hopkins Hospital, listing many striking examples, included the case of a doctor who experimented on patients with bleeding peptic ulcer, and *"70 percent showed excellent results lasting over a period of one year,"* when the doctor gave them an injection of distilled water, and assured them it was a new medicine that would cure them. A control group, on the other hand, *"who received the same injection from a nurse, with the information that it was an experimental medication of undetermined effectiveness showed a remission rate of only 25 percent,"* which suggests that if the medical profession had been content to exploit suggestion throughout, ulcer patients would have done better during the last fifty years than they have from all the treatments tried—a verdict now gaining official acceptance.*

The problem is not in the existence or nonexistence of the individual's self-healing powers, but in how to mobilize

*Brian Inglis, *The Case for Unorthodox Medicine* (New York: Putnam, 1967), pp. 43–44.

them and bring them into play in the person's search for health.

There are, of course, no guarantees of success in recovering from cancer. We do not have any final answers. The holistic medicine approach does tend to mobilize the person's self-healing abilities. Sometimes this makes a crucial difference. Even where it does not stop the progress of the disease, it usually improves the quality of life in the time that the person has left. The story of a man named Charles, with whom I worked, illustrates the point.

Charles was short, heavyset, and forty-three years old. He was rather quiet and undemonstrative and always carefully dressed. I never saw him without a white shirt, tie, and conservative suit. He was married, with one child. His father had died of cancer of the brain at forty years of age and his paternal grandfather of the same condition at fifty-one. His mother's family history was nonsignificant; most of the family had died of heart conditions at fairly advanced ages. I first saw him on a routine interview of patients who came to the outpatient clinic. By the end of the hour interview we had found that we liked each other. He wanted to continue to explore and make some sense out of his life. We set up a schedule of psychotherapy sessions and worked together for nearly two years.

Charles was an engineer who worked on the design of light machinery for a large company. He "rather enjoyed" his work, but told me he had always wanted to get into the field of designing large installations. He was particularly interested in designing desalinization plants and felt that the need for these was going to increase markedly in the next century. He had an idea for designing these using natural climatic heat and photoelectric panels. Rather excitedly, he told me that no one seemed to have realized the implications of the fact that the greatest need for these plants was in tropical climes with a strong sun. He knew that this project would be a long, difficult job but felt that it would be a fascinating one. When I asked him why he had never attempted to get into this kind of work or even tried to convince his company of its validity, he looked at me silently. Finally he said: "I've been interested in this for dog's years, but I guess I never got around to doing anything about it."

In the middle of his forty-second year, he began to develop some strange symptoms. There were transitory anesthetic areas on his arms, and sometimes sensations would be changed; for example, something dull would feel sharp, and so forth. There were also a few falls and sudden losses of balance, inexplicable to him. These brought him to his physician, who sent him for a full neurological workup. A deep-seated brain tumor was diagnosed. Further studies showed it to be inoperable. The amount of radiation that would have been needed to be effective would have caused intolerable brain damage. No relevant chemotherapy was available at this time—the early 1970s. The prognosis was given as extremely negative.

In psychotherapy we began to discuss what Charles thought and felt about his life as a whole. He said, "My life is good and it's pleasant. I have everything I thought I'd have when I grew up. But I look around and say, 'Is this all there is?' I look at my life and I ask 'Why?' I enjoy myself mostly, but it all seems rather empty. There's no purpose, no *reason.*"

A few years before he had started to think about his life and given up hope of anything more. Up to then he had still, he told me, had his childhood dreams of "something great and wonderful. Something wow!" Now, however, he realized that those dreams were just fantasies and could never be fulfilled.

After we had worked in psychotherapy for a few months, he went to the director of his company and asked for an unpaid leave of absence (he needed this rather than leaving the job so he could keep up his insurance and medical benefits), while he worked on his desalinization ideas. The director asked him about these ideas. They talked about them for a whole after-

noon, and Charles was offered a paid year on a research assignment to see how the ideas progressed. He would have full use
of company facilities such as computer time, and the like, and
be on full salary. If his ideas worked out, they would belong to
the company, but he would recieve 25 percent of any profits
made on them.

As can be imagined, Charles was ecstatic. He had never
done anything like this before, really stood up for himself and
what he wanted. Instead he had "drifted" (as he put it), into a
major in college, his current job, and even his marriage. He was
startled at the positive result of his action now. In therapy he
began to examine carefully the reasons for his previous passivity.

Charles was very excited about the new work and found
that it was fascinating. He stopped being concerned about a lack
of meaning. He was in the midst of his life and actively engaged
in it. When we are actively singing our own song, we realize that
it is only philosophers and depressives who ask what is the
meaning of life. When we are using ourselves in the way we are
built for, we *know.*

When we began to explore his relationships with his wife
and child, we found that Charles had a long-term fear of too
much caring and of too much emotional involvement. This
seemed to us to have been conditioned largely by the death of
his father when he was nine years old. Charles strongly believed
that if he loved or cared about anyone too much, then that
person would be taken away and that he could not bear again
the flame of this kind of separation. As we worked through these
painful feelings, he relived the agony he had felt at his father's
death and the subsequent loneliness during the following years
when his father was hardly mentioned around the house and it
was as if he had never existed. He began to understand that this
had been his mother's way of handling her pain, and she had
never realized how much worse this had made it for him. During
this period he found that his relationship with his wife and
daughter deepened and became a much more powerful force in
his life. They began to share their anxiety over his cancer and
several times found themselves weeping together. With surprise

he told me that afterward they all felt better. "I always thought that if you talked about these things they got worse," he told me.

Charles began to search for an exercise and movement program that would be right for him. He finally settled on a stationary bicycle that he would ride for an hour a day while watching a late TV program. He found that he enjoyed this and felt better and more energetic in those weeks when he had exercised regularly than when he had not.

A nutritionist suggested a macrobiotic diet, but after trying it Charles felt that it was not right for him. It was not so much that he did not like the food as that after a period on this diet, he felt that it was doing him more harm than good. He listened carefully to the messages his body was giving him and quit the diet. He settled on a program of chicken, fish, and raw or undercooked vegetables. To him this diet felt valid, particularly when supplemented by vitamins and minerals. It seemed to him to increase his energy and his feelings of well-being. In addition, he lost some of the extra weight he had been carrying. No mainline medical program was available—just regular, routine neurological examinations.

Charles also began a regular meditation program. Six mornings a week he spent half an hour staying as awake and aware as possible and trying to do nothing but count his breaths. He tried to catch himself more and more quickly when he drifted off and his mind went somewhere else, and to bring himself back more and more firmly, gently, and lovingly. He reported that he felt better for doing this, and the few times he skipped the practice, he missed it and felt somehow "lacking in something" during that day.

Charles's concern with the present and future water needs of the world, and particularly the Third World countries, seemed to both of us to also be an expression of his spiritual needs.

For nearly a year there was no apparent change in his cancer. During this time he continued to work on his project. He felt that his life was fuller and richer than it had ever been and that no matter what happened, he was living his individual and own life to the full. Then the cancer started to show new symptoms. The anesthesias and paresthesias became more extensive and more frequent. Charles began to lose his balance more and more often. Then an aphasia appeared—he had increasing difficulty in finding the words to express his thoughts. He could think clearly but could not speak or write. He could not read, although he could understand someone else's speech. He also began to get weaker and weaker until he could not get out of bed. It was clear that he was dying.

The day before he died he tried desperately to communicate something to me. For over an hour he tried, working as hard as he could, but only jumbled words came out. He was terribly frustrated and kept trying until he fell back on his bed, exhausted. I saw him again that evening and the same scene was repeated until he collapsed in complete exhaustion. I could make no sense at all of the message he was trying so hard to give me. By the next morning he was dead.

For a long time I wondered what he had been trying to tell me. It seemed that this would be one of those mysteries that can never be solved. Then about five years ago I met his wife at a concert. We talked for a time during the intermission and met afterward for coffee. When I told her about the last two times I had seen Charles, she said, "Oh, I think I know what he wanted to say. Several days before he died, he told me that he knew that he hadn't been able to lick the cancer and was on his way out. He said that he was going to tell you that you had given him the gift of living and loving more fully at long last." I told her that I wished he had been able to say that, because then I could have told him that he had done it for himself.

7

MINIMIZING "BURNOUT" FOR ALL CONCERNED

During the first ten years of the work that resulted in this book, I worked entirely with patients who were medically considered to be "hopeless"—whose condition had not responded, and it was believed would not respond, to medical intervention. There were two reasons for working with these particular patients. The first was that I was exploring new territory and trying something new. I did not know what effect the work I was doing would have on the tumors' development. Any procedure that can have positive effects can also, at least theoretically, have negative effects if not used correctly, and there was no previous experience to guide me. Therefore, for ethical reasons, I could work only with patients whose condition was terminal and it was permissible to take chances. All patients were, of course, informed of this situation.

The second reason was that I worked in a cancer treatment center that was "a court of last resort." The Institute of Applied Biology largely served a cancer population whose cancer had not been arrested with radiation, surgery, or the chemotherapy that was known at that time.

While my therapy method was being developed, I had to

live with the fact that nearly all my patients died. At one time I made a count and found that of the forty-seven people with cancer that I had worked with for over one hundred hours, forty-seven had died. (This did not include the many people I worked with for shorter periods—nearly all of whom also died.) As I have never believed that it is possible to be an effective psychotherapist unless you are emotionally involved—unless you really *care* about the people you are working with and actively want the best for them—the effect on me was devastating. I was constantly in active mourning for people for whom I cared deeply.

In addition, I had built up a very heavy practice. The word as to what I was doing was on the hospital grapevine. I frequently received calls from patients asking me to work with them. When I replied that I was overloaded but could see them in six months, the answer would often be something like: "In six months I'll be dead!" And I would have more patients. At one point I was seeing patients for an average of ten hours a day!

The word *burnout* had not yet been invented and I was not aware of the concept. I therefore took no precautions against it. Finally one patient, a woman I loved very much, died. Suddenly I was completely drained and empty. I had nothing left to give, no emotional or relating energy left. I felt like a large barrel of water that had been emptied and now they were scraping the sides with pails trying to extract the last drop of moisture!

As far as my patients went, I became a walking disaster area. I made the same number of visits of the same length and said pretty much the same things as I had before, but there was no feeling left. For many of my patients, their worst fantasy was being fulfilled: as soon as they fully showed themselves to someone else, that person deserted them. I had not gone away physically, but I had emotionally, and they all felt it.

Although I did not fully comprehend what had happened, with the guidance of my control (supervising) psychotherapist, I at least had the sense not to take any new patients. Presently I had no patients, as all of the people I was working with had died.

I felt desperate and lost. I simply had to get away and be

completely by myself. I had never done anything like this before and no one close to me understood. I did not really understand it myself.

I chose a country I loved but whose language I did not speak at all—and went off to Greece, for six weeks. During that time I walked in the back country and avoided anyone who knew any English at all. I had absolutely no desire to communicate with anyone on any subject. It took that long for my "skin" to regrow and my reserves of relationship energy to be filled up. At the end of six weeks I was sitting in a taverna in Sparta in the evening of a long hot day. Two pretty American college girls sat down at a nearby table. When I looked at them and found myself saying "Hmm-mm," I knew I was cured and went home the next day.

I tell this story to illustrate how severe burnout can get. Since then I have seen it happen to many patients, family members, friends, and involved health professionals.

I remember one woman who was the mother of a daughter with severe leukemia. Elena was very good with the child—supportive, loving, always open to discussion and ready to talk with her on the big as well as the small questions, and making sure that she was encouraged to be as strong and independent as possible and was not smothered by other people's anxiety. The father was an army major who had been killed in Vietnam. There were no other children or close relatives. Elena received some emotional and physical support (including a part-time housekeeper) from Cancer Care, an organization that is set up to help with this type of problem and does it very well indeed. The strain on her was very great. She had to keep up her work as accountant and company comptroller to support the two of them. She reported that she was becoming more and more irritable on the job and beginning to make mistakes in her work. Her automobile driving was becoming erratic and she had several minor accidents after many years with a faultless driving record. Elena had been quite svelte and now had become thirty-five pounds overweight (at five foot two).

In our discussion, I told her that she was like the battery of a car in which there is no generator. She kept putting out and putting out and nothing was coming in. She was getting more and more emotionally exhausted and if she kept up like this would soon be no use to herself, her job, or, eventually, to her daughter. She would have to serve as her own generator. What did she most need to fill her, to help keep up her emotional supplies? I pointed out that the very fact that she paid attention to her own needs and took thought, care, and what time she could for herself in itself would be helpful.

What she needed most, Elena said, was sleep and some time off. For many and obvious reasons, it was impossible to take much time away from her work and home. We decided that she would take one weekend off at a hotel where they had room service. I arranged with her physician that she have a couple of sleeping pills so that she could take full advantage of the brief time. After that, one evening a week would be just hers. She would carefully plan these evenings—mostly what she felt would be most refreshing would be supper and a movie with a friend. Her friends had long since stopped calling her as she never had time for them. She would now call them and say that she was ready. In addition she would get up twenty minutes earlier each day and fill those twenty minutes with a physical exercise program.

Contrary to her expectations, paying attention to and being aware of her own needs and feelings did not weaken her, but had the opposite effect. Although her overall program and the pressures on her were the same as they had been, she became less irritable and stopped making mistakes at work. She had no more car accidents. She was able to continue doing what she had to until the daughter died three years later.

The concept of burnout has generally been applied to "helpers" and health professionals. It is not usually recognized that the suffering of cancer patients themselves can also be markedly increased by this condition. They also can suffer from burnout. Not only do the anxiety and fear, the physical discomfort and pain of living with cancer do this; the fact that the person with cancer is living in a waking nightmare has a weakening and exhausting effect.

There is a difference between a bad dream and a nightmare. A nightmare is a dream with three factors, all present:

1. Terrible things are happening and/or worse are threatened;

2. Your will is helpless to aid you—there is nothing you can do. Any hope resides in other forces or people (as in new medical discoveries about which you can have no real effect and on whose appearance your life depends); and

3. There is no time limit.

If any one of these three is not present, it is a bad dream. If all three are there, it is a nightmare with a nightmare's special ego-weakening and emotionally and physically exhausting effects.

The cancer patient wakes up each morning to a nightmare. Terrible things are happening or threatened. Everything rests not on his or her will, but on the medical profession. Living constantly in a nightmare frequently leads to severe burnout. And this is often made worse because it is unrecognized by others (after all, patients have no right to be exhausted—isn't everyone doing the best they can for them?) and patients do not accept the fact that it is a legitimate condition either (after all, patients are supposed to keep trying to get better and not to be too tired or discouraged. They are supposed to be able to keep up their recovering energy).

One of the most weakening factors in the cancer situation is the steady pressure to stop thinking and feeling about yourself as a person who happens to be sick at the moment and to start responding to yourself as a sickness that seems to have a person somehow attached to it. All your efforts and thoughts gradually get turned toward the illness and the treatment. They take up more and more of your time and energy.

One of the most exhausting aspects of an illness like cancer is the demand (of both others and ourselves) that we should always be responsible and calm and upbeat about the situation. Others around us, and we ourselves, demand that we always be well organized and hopeful. If the patient and family behaves in this way all the time, it is certainly easier on the health professionals involved but harder on the patient and his loved ones. To quote the philosopher Nietzsche: "Some situations are so bad that to remain sane is insane." If you have cancer (or if someone you love has it), it is only rational to be sometimes irrational about it; to go a bit crazy from time to time. Patients (and those very close to them) should allow themselves this—whatever form it takes for them—to take a holiday from always having to be in such good mental control. Families, friends, and professionals should relax and let this happen when it happens to a patient or to those very close. It is important not to let our anxiety overwhelm us and make us give in to the tendency to calm down and reassure the person and thereby reassert that it is not acceptable to have periods of simply giving way to feelings and saying the hell with calmness and rationality. If this happens sometimes, everyone will feel better later and it will *increase* control, not weaken it.

To avoid or lessen burnout, the person with cancer should develop a fierce and tender concern for *all* of the self, not just the physical, and be actively concerned with his or her psychological, emotional, and spiritual growth. This is not the time to let these go because we are concerned so much with the physical. It may seem to be only common sense to do this—to say that we have so much on our plate in the physical illness that everything else can and must be put off until another, more peaceful period. However, common sense often fails to be an adequate guide in areas where we do not have real experience. The opposite of what seems "reasonable" is true here. We strengthen ourselves by working hard on our growth and "becoming" when we are under the hammer of fate. It is a time to redouble our efforts.

If, however, we are going to redouble our efforts, we must be especially careful that we have not forgotten our aim. Where are we going with our life? What do we want out of it? Let's put this a different way. How can we make our life different and far better after the illness than it was before? How can we find the *context* within which we want to lead our life and guide our own *becoming*?

If there is a *goal* and a *context* to life, a way to work so that there is reason to believe that life after the illness will be different, more individual, reflecting more of our true self, unique, then there is a much greater chance that the immune system, the cancer-defense mechanism, will be able to work more effectively on the side of life. No other factor appears to me to be as crucial as the presence or absence of this.

In addition, of course, working toward a meaningful life goal changes the feeling of life very greatly. No more are we just reacting, helpless pawns in a struggle between the medical profession and death. We are actively fighting for our being, our soul. And, since this does help our physical being also, we have broken the nightmare condition. Our will is no longer helpless to aid us—we have found a way to fight for our life. As a nightmare requires that *all* three factors be present—terrible things are happening, your will is helpless, and there is no time limit—we are now living in a bad dream, not a nightmare. The change is very real. With a goal to our life, our ability to bear and handle the discomfort and pain is also increased. Nietzsche wrote: "Where there is a 'why,' we can bear any 'how.' "

There is one difference between the cancer health professional on the one hand and the patient, family, and involved friend on the other. For the professional this involvement is part of a way of life. It is not a temporary condition, but a permanent aspect of his or her life. In order to avoid burnout, professionals must consciously accept the same factors as apply to the patient as an integral part of their profession. Health professionals must have the same fierce and tender concern for all aspects of their being—the physical, the mental and emotional, and the spiritual. All must be consciously examined from time to time to determine which aspect is in the most need of upgrading *at this time.*

The context of the work must also be taken into conscious examination from time to time. Why is he or she doing it? Any answer that is not basically a selfish one should be regarded with suspicion. If it is just for "altruistic" reasons, then, in all probability, the person is fooling him- or herself. The lack of honesty with the self in this area is very likely to seriously hamper the work and prove damaging both to the self and to the patients.

Any psychotherapist working in this field should also have a control or supervising therapist—irrespective of the amount of experience and training he or she has had. I believe this to be true for all psychotherapists, no matter what kind of patients they have. I personally will not refer anyone to therapists who do not from time to time realize that they are out of their depth, that with a particular patient they do not know what they are doing, or that a patient is mobilizing their anxiety in a personality area on which they still have work to do. And who, in these situations, do not go to someone else for help for a time. In my opinion, any therapist who does not think that he or she needs guidance occasionally is a very poor therapist indeed. It is even more necessary when therapists work with cancer patients. Our own mourning and sadness for those who die, our anxiety about avoiding more pain and loss, the necessity of facing our own mortality and of being actively concerned on a long-term basis with the great questions of human existence and meaning—all these contribute to our need for the kind of clear self-examination that psychotherapy provides.

In addition, therapists must be consciously concerned about their own growth and becoming. They must keep involved with the process of becoming unique and individualized, of working toward the full flowering of the self. Unless they do this, they are saying to patients "Do as I say, not as I do." This saying makes the rest of their work seem hollow and false indeed and is *always* ultimately communicated to patients.

It goes without saying that every patient has the right to question how a therapist's theories can be applied to his or her own life. If the questions are not answered, there is always the door and another therapist somewhere in the neighborhood.

I do not believe that any therapist should have a full-time practice of people with cancer. There should be a strong leavening of other types of patients. Similarly, other professionals working in the field of catastrophic illness should have other interests that they are heavily invested in emotionally. Everything I have said here about the psychotherapist is also true to some extent for all the other health professionals involved. The oncology nurse, the hospital attendant, the hospice worker, the oncologist—and their patients—will all benefit from paying attention to these ideas.

All Dorothy's friends had marveled at how well she was taking her diagnosis and treatment. She had had a kidney cancer, and in the first surgery one kidney, her urethra, and part of her bladder were removed. For the first two years after the diagnosis she kept up her normal life as far as possible and continued her work as a curator in an art museum. In spite of the surgery and several long and debilitating courses of chemotherapy, innumerable medical appointments and tests, conferences with a nutritionist, and a complex diet, Dorothy managed to keep up her work, see friends, attend the theater, and even go on a short summer vacation to the mountains.

Dorothy had always wanted to be married and have a family. She loved children and had wanted to have several. She had been married for a year and a half. At the end of this time her husband had told her that he was not cut out for marriage, had been happier as a bachelor, and wanted a divorce. Since then she had lived alone. The cancer was diagnosed one and a half years after the divorce.

After the first two years of cancer treatment, Dorothy became more and more tired and found it harder and harder to keep up with life. She gradually stopped seeing friends, going out in the evenings, and so forth.

At that time I was interviewing every fourth patient who came through the clinic in order to make sure that the patients I had been seeing in depth were a fair cross-section of the patients who came for treatment. Dorothy told me how tired she felt: "I just have no more energy. Life has become so *dreary* and exhausting. All I do is pay attention to my body. If I'm not running my blender or growing sprouts (or eating the tasteless things), I'm going to another doctor's office or lying under another X-ray machine. I feel like this is all I'll be doing for the rest of my life. For the first two years I could do it. I'm a naturally optimistic person. I could keep going. Now I seem to *care* less and less. Life is all medical details, what did I eat today and how did I urinate yesterday and which doctor do I see next. I just don't have the energy to care about anything any longer."

There was a deep feeling of exhaustion about her. We talked awhile about activities that would refresh her, about support groups, and so forth, but clearly she did not have the energy to take any action in those directions. Six months later further metastases were discovered. These progressed very rapidly and she died shortly after her admission to the hospital.

8

THE PERSON WHO IS DYING

It is a sad fate for a man to die too well known to everybody else and still unknown to himself.

—FRANCIS BACON

First, a caution. This chapter, more than any of the others, is directed toward the psychotherapist who is working with people who are dying. If you yourself are in the Dying Time, or if you are closely involved with someone who is, this chapter may be well worth reading. But if you are a family member or close friend, do not try to become a psychotherapist. Maintain and deepen the role and relationship you have; do not take another one that not only do you not have the training for, but one that is likely to weaken your present relationship and deprive the dying person of an important source of support and nourishment.

See what in the chapter speaks to you and what does not. You may find it useful to discuss some of the ideas with the dying person or use them in whatever way fits both of your personalities and helps move your relationship toward its fullest potential for mutual richness.

A man came to consult with me once. His father was dead and his mother was dying of cancer in a hospital. Sal was the only child who went to visit her regularly. But he did not know what to say to her. They both knew that she was dying, and their pattern of talk of the trivia of his and her everyday life seemed extremely unsatisfying. Sal *wanted* to relate to her more and to somehow help her more at this parting time, but he had no idea as to how to go about this. The daily visits were becoming more and more dreary and depressing times in which they sat and looked at one another, held hands with nothing to say, and felt increasingly frustrated.

After talking with him for a time and getting a sense of what was occurring in his life (recognizing, for example, that there did not appear to be a hidden agenda that was blocking communication), I asked Sal how much he knew about his mother's childhood. When he told me that he knew very little, I said that this was the last chance he would ever have to find out about her roots as well as his own. What had her early years been like? Her young life? What had been the most exciting period of her whole life? What major decision had been the best of her life? What had been the worst? In short, who was she and what life had she led? These would be important memories after she died. He would be someone who still had knowledge and the understanding of her. And he could pass this on to his children.

We talked in this vein for some time. Then Sal left. A month later he came back to see me again. He had just come from the funeral. Everything had changed after he had seen me. The next afternoon when he had gone to the hospital, he had begun to ask his mother about her childhood. She had been surprised and wanted to know why he was so interested. He answered: "Because I love you and there is so much I don't know about you. I want to know about your life and when I have children, I want to be able to tell them about you. What was a young girl's life like in 1915 when you were growing up?"

The visits changed. There now seemed so much to talk

about, so much to explore together. Mostly they talked about her and her life, but in the discussions Sal was able to tell her things about his own life that he had never shared with her. As they exchanged ideas and memories, both felt richer. She became more and more interested, not only in telling him about her life but in exploring it for herself. Frequently she would say things about her own life such as "I never thought of it in that way before" or "So that was what that was all about." When he came into the hospital room, there were many fewer complaints about the nurses, the food, and the doctors. Rather she had an active and excited sense of exploration.

After a few visits of this sort, he brought in a tape recorder. She taped her recollection of special events in her own life, some stories for the future grandchildren, and descriptions of her own parents and grandparents. One day she asked him to leave the tape recorder with her overnight. The next day she told him that she had taped a message to him to be listened to after her death. He played it the night before her funeral. In it she expressed her thanks and gratitude to him for changing her whole dying experience.

About five hours before she died, Sal told me, there had been a change in her whole personality. "She seemed to light up from within. She became very calm and serene. Yes, that's the word, serene." When the nurse came with her usual pain medication, she said that she did not need it. "She was calm, relaxed, and seemed somehow happier than I have ever seen her."

She said good-bye to him, gave him a few messages—of forgiveness and peace and good wishes for some relatives and friends—and then closed her eyes and died.

In this case, a patient I never saw directly accomplished the three goals necessary in working with the person in the Dying Time. The last period of life changed color. It turned into a time of active growth and becoming, where the patient began to view the whole of her life and see it as a *Gestalt,* an integrated pattern. She died a transcendent death. The family was left with as little emotional scarring as possible.

Some time ago I attended a lecture on psychotherapy for people who have a catastrophic illness. The speaker pointed out, quite correctly, that this concept includes two separate types of therapy. In the first, we are dealing with people who are in the sick mode. For these, the primary problem is how to get well again and, if possible, in this process, set up the situation so that the illness will be less likely to recur. In the second type of therapy, the patient is in the dying mode. Here the goals are entirely different.

The speaker went on to say that there are people in the field who specialize in one aspect of the therapy and people who specialize in the other. For example, he said, there is a Dr. X who is a specialist in helping people to die. His vision is entirely in this direction. He typically comes into a hospital room in which there is a patient who has had a mild skin cancer that has been completely taken care of and who, unless hit by a truck, will probably live for many years and then die of old age. Dr. X comes in as the patient is getting dressed to go home and begins to help him or her get ready to die. Among other things, Dr. X asks about how he or she *really* feels about saying good-bye to loved ones.

On the other extreme, said the speaker, is Larry LeShan. (I began to listen with extra care at this point!) Typical of LeShan, he said, is his leaning over the bed, grasping the patient firmly by the shoulder, and asking "But what do you *really* want out of life?" At the same time, the nurse is pulling on his coattails and saying "But, Dr. LeShan, this patient died three hours ago!"

There is, unfortunately, some truth in this. (And, I might add, some exaggeration!) All of us who work with cancer patients are guilty of sometimes brutalizing patients by either being unable to recognize that they have moved from the sick to the dying mode or else by treating them as dying when they are in the sick mode. In order to avoid this brutalization, therapists must be aware of their own special orientation, compensate for it, and be as sensitive to patients as possible. As this is very often a difficult decision to make, a decision full of intangibles and arousing all sorts of feelings within the therapist, having a control therapist is particularly useful here. Discussing the problem with someone who is not personally involved is often very helpful—especially when a patient with whom you have been working in the sick mode may have shifted into the dying mode. Deciding when this occurs is particularly difficult for the therapist.

Each therapist will have to have his or her own ways of evaluating the moment when a patient shifts from the sick to the dying mode. One way I have found useful for myself is the appearance of a deep fatigue, a fatigue so profound that it appears to be the psychological equivalent of adrenal exhaustion. The patients literally have no more energy with which to fight for life. They have run the race, done everything possible, and have absolutely no more energy with which to continue. The exhaustion is basic and total. They desire only to rest.

> I am tired of tears and laughter
> And men who laugh and weep.
> Of what may come hereafter
> For men who sow to reap.
> I am tired of days and hours,
> Blown buds and barren flowers
> Desires and dreams and powers
> Of everything but sleep.
>
> From too much love of living,
> From hope and fear set free,
> We thank with brief thanksgiving
> Whatever Gods may be
> That no man lives forever,
> That dead men rise up never;
> That even the weariest river
> Winds somewhere safe to sea.
>
> —A. C. SWINBURNE, "The Garden of Proserpine"

Or, as the poet W. E. Henley described someone in this situation:

> *Tired of experience, he turns*
> *To the friendly and comforting breast*
> *Of the old nurse, Death.*

I have written of what the task of psychotherapy is when the patient is in the sick mode. What is the task when the patient is in the dying mode?

The psychotherapist working with people with catastrophic illness has (as does the physician in his or her practice) three tasks:

1. To cure where possible;
2. To alleviate where cure cannot be accomplished; And,
3. When neither of these can be done, to give safe passage. What does this last phrase mean?

Here again is a task that each therapist will have to define for him- or herself. Each will have to answer the question: What are we trying to accomplish when we work with people in their Dying Time? I can give only my own goals. They are threefold.

1. To change the color of the Dying Time so that for each person it is an exciting and interesting adventure in growth. So that it is not a dreary, depressed, or drugged time, but wherever possible, it is a *becoming,* a growth time, a full moving into the last task each of us will face, to die as well, as *completely,* as unafraid as possible. To know and warmly accept who we are before we die.

2. To help as many patients as possible achieve a "transcendent death."

3. To work toward a death that will leave the family with as little scarring as possible.

All three tasks are, I believe, best accomplished with the same approach.

Carl Jung wrote a story that is appropriate here. He had a patient, a woman in her mid-forties, who came to him for analysis. Midway in the analytic work, her husband's firm transferred him to a distant city and the therapy was broken off. Jung heard nothing more of her for many years. Then he received a call from a local hospital. They had a patient, they told him, a woman who was dying. She was also psychotic, seemed to recognize no one, talked constantly in meaningless sequences. Her family said that she had once been Jung's patient. He went to his files and took out the notes he had made years before when they were working together. When he approached her bedside she did not seem to recognize him, but went on verbalizing apparently meaninglessly. As Jung listened, her ramblings began to make sense. Through free association she was finishing the analysis that had been broken off so many years before! Jung stayed with her for two weeks while she finished the process and came to peace with the problems that had plagued her all her adult life. After finishing, she became lucid, recognized Jung, and greeted him. She remained calm, serene, and lucid until she died shortly afterward.

All of us need to understand before death the meaning of our lives. What was it all about? We need to consider ourselves in the last days not as being overwhelmed by disease, dying helplessly in a narrow and sterile hospital room, but rather as part of a tapestry of life or symphony in which all the parts interact with each other and our life is an integrated, rich, and varicolored whole.

We cannot really say good-bye to something without knowing what it was. Trying to give up, say farewell to, renounce our lives before fully accepting them, tends to lead to a death that is bitter and sad.

The essence of the task of the Dying Time is to see the whole of our lives as a pattern and a symphony in which the themes swell and recede and the whole makes a real and organic whole. It calls for fully forgiving and accepting ourselves, so that at the end we are real to ourselves, and not—as so many of us are to ourselves during our lives—a ghost to ourselves.

When the therapist focuses on this task as the real one for this developmental stage of patients' lives, when the therapist *means* that this is the valid and basic purpose of this time, then patients also can become engaged with it. And when patients become so involved, the color of the Dying Time changes. No longer are they helpless pawns, harried and wounded by the disease, driven helplessly out of life. The Dying Time then becomes the last adventure, an adventure as great as any others that patients have experienced. It becomes a time of growth and development.

In order to work with people in this period, therapists must be aware of something that all psychotherapists should know but rarely do. This is the fact that the laws of consciousness are closer to the laws of art and magic than they are to the laws that govern machines. Thus *honesty* on the part of the therapist is as much an observable, is as real, as *mass* or *inertia* are in the world of machines. Therapists cannot pretend belief or interest. It must be real or it damages the process and a person in the extremely vulnerable Dying Time. You can fake liking a Chevrolet and do as effective a job changing tires as you would if you really had a great deal of affection for the car. This is simply not true with people in their Dying Time. You cannot, repeat *not*, fake it. You can only do damage.

For example, soon I am going to give a number of sample questions of the sort you might use with dying persons in this period of their lives to help them start thinking about the meaning and structure of their lives. Unless you are *really* interested in the answers to these questions and are ready to stay with the persons and listen seriously, it is simply not permissible to ask them. To raise questions of this sort and then not to carefully listen to the answers is asking people in a very vulnerable and delicate life period to be open to themselves and then to walk away when they do.

In listening, you must learn not to reassure. What the dying persons need is someone to hear who they are and what their life is and has been. It is very easy to be reassuring—very easy and useless. Most professionals have learned this lesson well in working with patients in their living mode. We do not say to a depressed patient "You have a great deal to live for." We have long since learned that this is useless and only tells the patient that we have not really listened, that we have heard only the words and not the feeling and the life behind it. Although we have learned this with patients in the sick mode, we tend to forget it when we are with patients in the dying mode. Our anxieties become so great that we stop accepting where patients are and start to reassure them that they should not be there. This is easy to do and reduces the therapist's anxiety.

Below, I list a number of questions that can be helpful when working with people in the dying mode. These are *examples*, not techniques or gimmicks. Any serious relationship, and this hopefully includes psychotherapy sessions, must develop on its own terms if it is going anywhere beyond a ritual. There is no "right thing" for the therapist to do or say under this or that condition. (Remember those useless child-raising books that used to be so popular? They were full of statements like: "When the child says, ——" "The parent should respond ——" and then give the exact words.) This cannot occur when talking about psychotherapy. In fact, if there is a single rule, if there is one law in psychotherapy, it is "Miale's Law,"* which goes as follows: "Any response of the therapist that comes from techniques rather than from human feelings is antitherapeutic." The good therapist seeks to have a large—and constantly increasing—store of techniques and methods in his or her apperceptive mass, in the storehouse of memory, but uses them only when they rise to consciousness in an appropriate context—when they come "trippingly on the tongue" and feel to both the therapist and the patient to be completely spontaneous. It is not only that the sophistication level with which the question or technique is framed must be appropriate to the patient. The question or technique itself must be a natural outgrowth of what is going on in the sessions at that moment. If not, the relationship is reduced to a mechanical interaction that is useless in furthering and nourishing the patient's growth and becoming.

*The rule was formulated in this way by Florence Miale, Ph.D., a New York City psychotherapist.

What kind of statements and questions are useful in helping patients toward the task appropriate in the Dying Time? How can we work with patients to help them begin to search for the meaning of their lives; to look for the patterns and the themes that made them unique; to look for what was their real name and what helped and what hindered them from living under it?

The questions that follow are suggestions to stimulate the imagination, to help the therapist, relative, or close friend see some of the ways that this last task can be approached. They should not be used as a list to be read to the patient, but rather they are an album of sketches, deliberately put in no particular order, of some of the roads that might lead us in the direction of growth in the last days. Each person using them will have to change and color the sketches to fit his or her personality and the special and unique relationship that exists at this moment.

Some of these questions may sound quite sophisticated and too advanced for many people. I can only say, on the basis of long experience with a wide variety of people in their Dying Time, that, if phrased with some respect for the background of the person you are with, if they are appropriate to the relationship right now, if there is real interest on the questioner's part, that the very great majority of people in this period of their lives respond to them as they would to an unexpected oasis found in the desert.

1. As you look at your whole life from the viewpoint of where you are now, what was it all about? Was it a good life? Was it a lonely life? Was it a frustrating life?

2. If your whole life had been designed in advance so that you would learn something from it, what would be the lesson you were supposed to have learned? Did you really learn it? What else would you have needed in order to have learned it?

3. What was the best thing that ever happened to you? What was the worst? (These are separate questions and, as a general rule, seem to be the most helpful whan asked in this order.)

4. What was the best thing you ever did? What was the worst?

5. What was the best period of your life? What was the worst?

6. How would you finish these statements: "Out of my childhood I love to remember . . ." "Out of my childhood I hate to remember . . ."?*

7. Do you believe it to be true that "It is better to have loved and lost than never to have loved at all?" What led you to this conclusion?

8. If you were asked by a child you love to tell him or her the one most important thing that you have learned in life, what would you reply?

9. There is an old Greek legend about the three Fates who govern all lives: Clotho, who weaves the thread of a person's life; Lachesis, who colors it; and Atropos, who cuts it and the person dies. How did Lachesis color *your* life? Did Atropos cut it too soon? Too soon for what? Can you still do what you have unfinished so far?

10. In each symphony (ballad, folksong, popular song) there is a central theme. It has many variations, these appear in the different sections (verses), but underlying them all is the theme. What has been the theme of your life?

11. If you could change *one decision* of your life, what would it be? Why did you make it the way you did? What does this tell

*This question was suggested by family-life psychologist Jean Schick Grossman.

you about how you saw yourself and the world at that time? Can you forgive yourself for making that decision the way you did? For feeling the way you did? If not, why not?

12. For the things you did, what do you now need to do in order to be able to forgive yourself?

13. For the things that others did to you, what do you need to do in order to forgive them? For the things that happened to you, what do you need in order to forgive yourself?

14. If you were to overhear your friends talking about you at your funeral, what would you most like to hear them say about you? Like least to hear?

15. As you look back at your life, what were the moments when you were most yourself? What helped you to do this? What were the moments when you were least yourself? Why do you think this was so?

16. What was the best time of your life? Tell me about it. What was the worst time of your life? Tell me about it.

17. How were you the same all your life, as a child, a youth, an adult, now? How were you different at these different times of your life?

18. What do you need to finish your life, to complete it? Can you do it from this hospital room?

19. During this time, what is the longest time of day for you? What do you mostly feel and think during this time?

20. In an ancient manuscript *The Book of Splendor* is the statement: "God's purpose is not to add years to your life, but to add life to your years." What do you think of this?

21. What is the thing in yourself that you have been most afraid to experience consciously? To think and feel about? Does it now seem as necessary to hide it from yourself as it did in the past?

22. What is it about you that you have most hidden from others? Does it seem as necessary to keep it hidden as it did in the past?

23. All our lives we try to change people to what we think that they should be. At this time of life we can often see that love is accepting people as they are and letting them be while hoping and wishing for more for them. Can you do this with those you love? What in you keeps you from this?

24. The time of dying is the last learning time we have on Earth. What lesson is there for you to learn in your dying? What in you keeps you from being able to learn it?

25. What is the major role that you have played in recent years? What masks have you worn most often in the presence of others? Are they roles you wish to play during these last times?

26. All our lives we try to *accomplish* something, to *do* something. What is it that you were trying to do in recent years? Is it still so important to you? How can you finish the attempt so that it ends with the most harmony and honesty?

27. Have you been mostly walking one road in recent years? Is there another road that you now need to walk in order to make your life journey more complete?

28. Is there someone you protected in recent years at a high cost in energy and time? Are you still trying to protect him or her? (Or be something for him or her?) Is it the best thing for this person for you to continue protecting him or her? For you?

29. What do you need to *finish* your life? Can you do it from this bed? How or why not? It is in *you* that we need to finish things and it is inside yourself that you can.

> I never saw a moor,
> I never saw the sea.
> But still I know what the heather is
> And what a wave must be.
>   EMILY DICKINSON, No. 1052

30. What is it that has happened to you that you have never been able to forgive God (or the Fates) for?

> Oh, Thou who man of baser earth did make,
> And even in Eden did devise the snake,
>   For all the sins wherewith the face of man is blackened,
> Man's forgiveness give—and take!
>   The Rubáiyát of Omar Khayyám

31. For what do you most need the forgiveness of God?

32. There is the story of one of the great Hasidic Rabbis named Zusya. His congregation asked him to do something, a particular political action. He refused. They said, "If Moses were our Rabbi, he would do it." Zusya answered, "When I die and rise and stand before the throne, God will not ask me why I was not Moses. He will ask me why I was not Zusya." Does this story in any way relate to you and your life? How?

33. What has been the best season of the year for you? Why?

These questions may seem to be asking a great deal of the dying person and to be suggesting that a very large amount of growth—growth that in other periods of life would take years of living and/or psychotherapy to accomplish—is possible in a short period during the Dying Time. This is true. It is also true that this sort of growth is the *appropriate developmental task* of this period of life and thus can often be accomplished very rapidly.

The central and critical question with which we approach people in their Dying Time is something to the effect: "How do you feel about what is happening to you?" This says (if it is really meant as a question that you want an answer to) "We can talk about anything you wish. I am not afraid. I am not a part of the conspiracy of silence that surrounds you unless you wish me to be." The people are given an open situation that is not assaultive or demanding. They can respond in any way, from complaints about the food or the nursing care to sorrow about leaving loved ones or grief over an unlived life or fear of an after-life. The amazing thing about this question is how rarely it is asked.

Sometimes the dying person responds merely to superficial aspects of the dying situation. The questioner may feel that the patient wants to speak of other things but does not quite yet trust the fact that the questioner is really, if implicitly, saying "I will and can talk about anything you wish. Your agenda is my agenda." In this case the following two questions also are very nonassaultive and, at the same time, convey the message: "What is the longest part of the day for you now? What occupies your mind during this time?"

> In the middle of the night things well up from the past that are not always cause for rejoicing—the unsolved, the painful encounters, the mistakes, the reasons for shame or woe. But all, good or bad, painful or delightful, weave themselves into a rich tapestry, and all give me food for thought, food to grow on.
>
> —MAY SARTON, *At Seventy*

A second, often useful, exploratory question is: "If you could change one part of what is going on now—not the overall result, but one part—what would it be?

The dying person is saying a multitude of different good-byes. By being sensitive to and comprehending these different farewells, therapists and friends can help the dying person accomplish the dying work. When you are in the Dying Time, you are leaving:

1. Yourself: Your own being, your pains and sufferings, your hopes and aspirations, the things accomplished and the things left unfinished.

2. Those parts of yourself that you left unfulfilled up to now; those parts neither watered by full recognition nor nourished by acceptance and expression. This is the last chance to recognize them, greet them warmly in passing, and—at long last—integrate them with the rest of your being.

3. Those you loved and the unfulfilled possibilities in you of loving them more and of more fully recognizing their love for you. In Elizabeth Barrett Browning's sonnet, "How do I love you . . ." she lists many ways of loving, from "the depth and breadth and height my soul can reach" to "the level of every day's most quiet need by sun and candlelight." These ways, those we have experienced and depths of loving that have never been reached before can now be had and experienced.

4. Those people that you have unfinished business with. Unless your affairs with them are now finished, they never will be and your death will be that of a person torn in two directions, toward life and toward death, and therefore be difficult, unpeaceful, and that of a wounded animal.

5. That general nature of which we are all a part. It is the last chance to learn the solace and heartwarming and heartfilling quality of loving, appreciating, and paying attention to the beauty of nature. In a medieval story a monk stopped to listen to the song of the bird. He listened completely, and when he resumed his journey, found that one hundred years had passed by.

Something we have known for many years is of deep importance in comprehending the world of the dying person. This is the fact that without purpose, without meaning, the inner life decays. We need a goal to keep our being intact. There is a truth in the biblical saying "Where there is no vision, the people perish" (Proverbs). Whether put in these terms or in Hegel's "Life has value only when it has something valuable as its object," we are saying the same thing. The dying person usually has no more goals to work toward. Even the close relationships which can themselves give our life meaning often are attenuated as the subject of loss and death is not one that most people can talk about easily. These are the central topics in the room, but they are generally not mentioned because each person involved is trying to "spare" the others. Yet this leaves them more vulnerable and lonely. The loneliness of the dying process can be very great and fill all existence; e. e. cummings described ". . . a smooth round stone as small as a world and as large as alone."

While facing one of the greatest crises of their lives, dying people are frequently in situations that weaken their ego and lessen their ability to solve relevant problems and take advantage of developmental opportunities. This is to say nothing of the fact that it is so very much harder for people in this weakened state to bear with the problems of fear, loneliness, regret, and loss.

The therapist or caring other solves this added difficulty by providing a goal that can and should be worked toward during the Dying Time. Comprehending the pattern and meaning of one's life is indeed a "something valuable"; is indeed a worthwhile and important goal and is very often so perceived by the dying person, irrespective of education or social class. The great majority of Westerners I have worked with in their Dying Time seem ready to explore the pattern of their lives.

Once dying people have a goal that engages them, the total situation changes. The decay of the inner life stops and reverses. Their mood is now different; the "helplessness" is no longer so prominent a feature. As Elizabeth Barrett Browning wrote:

Let no man until his death
Be called unhappy. Measure out the work
Until the day's out and the labor done.

Lying flat in the bed, unable to get up, fastened and made immobile by a catheter and assorted tubes and wires, people are often still able to engage in an active quest for the thing that—in the last analysis and when everything is said and done—is our ultimate concern, the growth of our own being. Or, if you will, the development of our soul. Most people are not aware that this is an important concern of theirs. Yet most are capable of finding this out in the last days if they have caring and concerned help.

——————— ▬ ———————

Aline was very much alone in the world. Her husband, parents, and siblings had all died in Ravensbrück concentration camp. She was the only physician in a small town and much loved by the people there. Her room was always full of flowers and cards from her patients and from the town council. But she was alone, not only because she had no family, but because she was so separate from much of herself.

In her late fifties, she lay in the hospital bed with a rapidly progressing pancreatic cancer. She hated herself for what she regarded as her failure in life "for not being a real doctor and reading the latest journals and taking special courses during my vacations. The journals mostly bored me so much that I would fall asleep or go outside and work in the garden after ten minutes. When one of my patients had a special problem I could look up the latest and newest treatment, but I never liked medicine. And I couldn't stand the meetings of the County Medical Society. I'd always find an excuse not to go."

During our work while she was in the sick mode, the following interchange took place.

> i: Isn't it time you started being concerned about you, and
> stopped being concerned about people's reactions to
> you?
>
> ALINE: But they're important. That's our job. What I have
> to do.
>
> i: Sometimes one's job is to cultivate one's own garden.
> The garden in one's backyard, or in the front, or the one
> in one's heart.
>
> ALINE: What's the use of cultivating a little patch of rocks
> surrounded by high thick hedges?
>
> i: That's how you see your heart?
>
> ALINE: Yes.

We worked together for some months. The cancer kept progressing. Aline became weaker and weaker, and it was apparent
that she had very little energy left with which to fight for her life.
She began to talk more and more about how it was now time
for her to die. One night she dreamed that she was standing on
a ledge outside the window on a high floor of a building. She
had been going to jump but had changed her mind. However,
it was too late. She was going to fall. There was nothing she
could do. Then "someone" reached out a hand to her from the
window. "I tried to reach your hand, but it was too late. I started
to fall."

We talked for several days about how she felt. We agreed
that it was time for her to go and shifted our approach from
fighting for her recovery to working toward her death—to doing
the dying work. We began to explore who Aline had to forgive
before she could die as a complete person. She had, she felt, to
forgive the little girl she had been and herself now for not having
been what she should have been. All her life she had loved
nature and beauty—she almost spat out "flowers and poetry!"—
when what was the right and real thing to care about was science
and helping other people. As a child she believed that she was

not a good person because of her likes and dislikes. She had studied philosophy and hated it but believed that she *should* have liked it.

When I asked her to recall the best moment of her life (the moment when she had felt richest and most at home with herself, the moment that showed what she was capable of feeling; if she could recover that sense of herself and the world, she could use that feeling when it was time to ride out of life), she told me about a time she had taken a vacation on the moors in Devon. "One afternoon I went for tea to a country inn. It was served outside in the most beautiful garden I have ever seen. I was surrounded by flowers of all kinds so perfectly arranged— the small ones in front, the medium-tall ones, then the great roses as a background. The colors were blended as if by God Himself. The bushes were full of singing birds. I sat in at a table in the center of the garden and my eyes were drunk with perfect beauty. I just sat there ecstatic, drinking it all in until I couldn't tell the colors from the scents from the sounds. It was a perfect moment. I never even noticed the famous Devon tea with clotted cream and homemade preserves." When I quoted to her from D. R. Gurney's "God's Garden"

> The warmth of the sun for pardon,
> The sounds of the birds for mirth;
> One is nearer God's Heart in a garden
> Than anywhere else on Earth.

she nodded and said seriously and quietly, "And nearer to my heart too."

At another time I asked her what her best season of the year had always been. She answered without hesitation that it was the spring and quoted to me part of Swinburne's poem about April, when

> . . . time remembered is grief forgotten
> And frosts are slain and flowers begotten,

And in green underwood and cover
Blossom by blossom the spring begins.

She felt she had been most nearly herself in a bird sanctuary in southern France in which she had once spent a week. "And in that garden in Devon I loved so much."

Gradually Aline developed compassion for the little girl who was taught—by well-meaning and loving parents who never dreamed how much they were hurting her—to reject her natural way of being and to take on—to please those she loved—an alien way of life. We agreed she was "a gardener manqué" and smiled together over this. Her smile was tender and thoughtful.

The central theme of her life had been that of a simple person trying to be herself in a world that rejected what she was. In her world, the only real value came from intellectuals who helped other people, and Aline had always agreed with this. This view was so reinforced by the people she met in college and medical school, by her experiences in the concentration camp, and by the love and respect she got from her patients that she had never questioned it. She had only blamed herself for not being able to enjoy enthusiastically the kind of life she had chosen. She felt that she *knew* this proved that there was something basically and profoundly wrong with her.

In spite of this, Aline had constantly expressed her real being in many ways. "Such as the place I chose for my practice. I picked a small town where I could have flowers and trees in my backyard and they liked the idea of my having my own herb garden. It fit with their old-country traditions. And in where I took my vacations. Always in places of nature." She further expressed it in the ordered beauty of the routines she had built in her life, a beauty she was only now beginning to understand.

"I guess I used my intelligence to fulfill both sets of needs—mine and my parents' for me. I was able to do both—to make them proud of me and find the beauty I needed. When you come right down to it, I wove it all together pretty well. I had my cake and ate it also. I don't see any way that anyone—no matter how intelligent she was or how hard she worked—could have made a better life out of such disparate elements. It was a pretty harmonious synthesis, wasn't it?"

About this time Aline rewrote her will. I was one of the witnesses at the signing and she later asked me to read it. Originally she had left all her money to the local medical society. "Now I'm not leaving them anything. I never liked those people or their pompous, self-absorbed meetings." Instead, she now divided her estate between the Sierra Club (an ecology organization) and the Simon Wiesenthal Foundation (an organization devoted to finding former Nazis and former concentration camp guards) "so that what happened to my parents and me will be less likely to happen again." About the will, she said, "I'm making this decision for me and it is *all* my decision. Maybe it's the first time in my life I've ever done that." Remaking the will was a brave statement on her part. It frightened her to do it, but she said, "It makes me feel proud."

The cancer was progressing and we were reaching the end. We decided to have a ceremony for her and the ending of her life. Aline chose music she wanted to hear for the last time, the last section of Haydn's *The Creation* and Mozart's Concerto for Four Horns. We filled her room with flowering plants and placed all the cut flowers she had in the room as background to them, took out the telephone, and I talked to the floor nurses to ensure privacy and hung up a DO NOT DISTURB sign. We played the music, said the Kaddish together for her parents, and she read, aloud at first and then to herself, some poetry in German that she had loved as a child. She then leaned back and recalled to herself again the experience in the garden in Devon and a garden she had played in as a child. After the ceremony she seemed to be serene and relaxed and to drift off to sleep. An hour later the nurse came in with her pain medication and she awoke, smiled, and told the nurse that she did not need it anymore. She went back to sleep and I left. She remained serene and calm with no need for the pain medication until the next afternoon when she died in her sleep.

Of course death work (or any other form of therapy) does not always end this well. However, this vignette shows the direction of the work and how it must be individualized to each patient so that each can comprehend and accept him- or herself.

Those who work with persons in the Dying Time should be especially aware of situations when it is widely said of a dying patient "He is taking it very well, isn't he?" This means that the dying person is showing no signs of how important the end of his life is; that he is being very careful not to upset anyone around him and is being protective of everyone else at a time when there are other things to be doing; that he is acting as if he were still in the sick role. To take this role in the last days is the person's inalienable right, and *no one* has the right to push him or her to change the way he or she chooses to spend the last days. But—and it is a very large *but*—most of the time that patients choose this role, it is not because they prefer to, but because they believe that it is what the hospital demands of them and that it is the way they are supposed to be. Very often when patients who have shown this kind of behavior are offered communication on their real feelings in such a way that it is plain that there is a real choice and they can freely choose, the behavior changes to a remarkable degree: the deep feelings so typical of this period are accepted by the patient and communicated and the patient is no longer in the usual position of the dying that Tolstoi described as "In the bosom of his family he was more alone than if he had been on the other side of the moon or at the bottom of the sea."

One major reason that a great many professionals do not wish to work with the dying and that relatives and friends are so uncomfortable with them is that they know they will not be able to answer many of the questions posed to them. Questions such as "Why me?" "What happens after death?" or "Why is life so unfair—whether you live or die bears no relationship to what kind of person you are."

Yet it is a mistake to believe that you—professionals or friends—are supposed to be able to answer these questions, that your image and the person's attitude toward you demand that you have a ready answer. This is very far from the truth. You are supposed to *hear* the questions and to understand that the patient is struggling with them. You can identify them as some of the great questions that humanity has always struggled with and say that some people find an answer and some do not, but that we humans have arrived at no *right* answer for everyone. The philosopher Emmanuel Kant wrote that there is a certain class of great questions that human beings are destined to have to face and be deeply concerned about, but that these questions could not—in principle, could not—be answered by logic or reason. They could only be answered personally by each person for him- or herself. One of us can provide clues or ideas for another, but never answers. The basic fact here is that the patient is not asking you to answer the question, but to hear it and comprehend its importance for him or her. A quick or a definitive answer will weaken your relationship far more than your giving no answer but just accepting where the patient is and what he or she is struggling with.

Working with the dying raises many anxieties that often block a therapist's ability to help the patient. Before anyone starts this work, I strongly recommend that, at the very least, you have a few therapy sessions yourself discussing your own feelings about your mortality. You may not be able to solve many problems in just a few sessions, but you will know more about your true feelings and so be able to compensate for them and prevent them from damaging the people you are trying to help.

Therapists working with the dying must expect that their patients will die! This sounds like a strange statement to make, but it is necessary. First, no matter how long the preparation, when someone we are emotionally involved with dies, we are not prepared. Death is too large and incomprehensible for us to deal with it in our usual terms. It is always a shock if we have been emotionally connected to the person.

This is not the place to go into detail about the therapist's feelings when a patient dies. Books such as Edgar Jackson's *Understanding Your Grief* have dealt with the matter in detail. But, briefly, therapists must expect themselves to react. These reactions will vary with the therapist, the relationship, and other variables, but they will be *real* and should be expected. They are not rational, they are not predictable.

Similarly, therapists should not expect rational or predictable reactions from relatives and friends of the person who died. From time to time they will be extreme and often in unexpected directions. Erich Maria Remarque told the story of three men he had known whose wives died suddenly in accidents. After the funeral, one went into his apartment, pulled down the shades, took out the phone, and spoke to no one for two weeks. The second went to his chess club and played steadily for two days until he fainted from exhaustion. The third went to the fanciest brothel in town, bought out the entire place, and had a weekend orgy. "I could never," said Remarque, "in my own mind, be sure which of these men loved his wife the most, or was the most wounded by her death."

In the usual hospital situation, there is tremendous pressure for dying patients to remain "good" patients and not make life difficult for the staff. The next time that you are on rounds in a service on which there are severely ill patients, stand back a bit and watch the body language of the medical staff as they unconsciously train patients how to respond and how a "good" patient responds. The doctor conducting the rounds asks something like "How do you feel today?" If the patient says, "I'm fine, Doctor, a bit better than yesterday," the physician keeps facing the patient, talks warmly with him or her for a moment, and *recognizes his or her existence* before turning back to the chart. If the patient says, "I'm much worse today, Doctor" (or even "I'm frightened that I'm dying" or "Why did this happen to me?") the physician turns body and attention away, toward the chart or toward some of the other staff with whom he discusses what medical procedures to do next and *ceases, as quickly as possible, to recognize the patient's existence.* This is indeed conditioning training—behavior modification with a vengeance.

It is true that many physicians do not behave in this way toward their patients. But a very large percentage do, and this includes some of the best, most competent, and most caring ones. They were trained to be most comfortable dealing with good patients, and unconsciously they train as many patients as possible to respond in "good" ways.

As very few professionals have been trained to relate to dying people, our anxieties make us retreat from them in ways of which we are often unaware. It is for these reasons that I repeat again that therapists who are going to work with patients with catastrophic illness *must* make clear efforts to know and accept how they themselves feel about this type of relationship.

During the time when Martha Gassmann, M.D., was my control (supervising) psychotherapist, we would meet regularly to discuss the cancer patients I was seeing. One day she said to me, "How is it going with Bobbie? You haven't mentioned her in some time."

I replied that Bobbie was doing fine and that I wanted to discuss problems with two other patients. Martha then said, "But first, let's spend a moment with Bobbie. How is *she* these days?" I responded angrily that she was fine and that I had important things to talk about this session. She said, "Yes, but for just one moment, how *is* she?"

At this point, I burst into tears. I realized that Bobbie was dying. We had worked together for a long time and I just had not been able to face what I knew was going on. I had withdrawn emotionally from her, fulfilling her worst fantasies that if she ever let anyone know who she really was, that person would reject her. I came into her room the right number of times and said all the right things, but emotionally I wasn't there and Bobbie knew it. I was making her Dying Time much worse.

The need for occasional supervision at least when working with the dying cannot be overstated. This is true no matter how experienced you are.

———————— ▬ ————————

There is a strong tendency (fortunately somewhat less every year) to give dying patients far more drugs than are necessary. I am not speaking here of drugs designed to control pain (these should be given in whatever amount is necessary), but of drugs designed to tranquilize the patient. Mostly this overmedication is due to the anxiety people in this mode give to the physican. First there is the strong possibility that unless discouraged by drugs they will ask questions that physicians mistakenly believe they should be able to answer. Second is the belief that dying patients reflect a failure of medicine and therefore of the doctor. This reflects the widespread twentieth-century Western superstition that *no one* dies unless medicine has failed to save him. Death is not seen as a natural conclusion to life but rather as due to inadequacies of the medical treatment. (In some primitive societies it is believed that *all* deaths are caused by hostile action of a witch, but of course these are very primitive societies!) Therapists working with people in the Dying Time should reflect on their own beliefs about this subject.

(There has certainly been a vast improvement in the past ten years as to how dying patients are treated in hospitals. We see much less, for example, of the use of heroic measures to the degree that the medical program becomes a long and hopeless torture before the person is allowed to die decently. Patients are more rarely being overwhelmed by extensive and useless surgical and chemical interventions.)

Sometimes the person goes into the dying mode much too early; they go into it when they have not yet exhausted their reserves nor found the potentialities within themselves which they can still garden. Early experience may have taught them that they cannot have nor express certain parts of themselves and yet these parts may still be ready for growth and fulfillment. It is the task of the therapist to be aware of this possibility.

Rae, a woman in her early seventies, was living in a Florida apartment house on the beach with her second husband. She had had four children, three of whom had died (one at Iwo Jima), as had her first husband. She had married right after high school, and all her life had been a housewife, taking care of two families. Now she, her husband, and all the other retired people of the apartment house spent their days sitting around the pool, talking about the television shows that they watched, playing cards, and planning whom to go out to dinner with that evening. Life for all of them was uneventful, physically easy, boring, and unfulfilling. Although some men and women in the building worked either at paid or volunteer jobs, very few of the others considered this possibility—despite the fact that those who worked had the highest status and were the most sought-after dinner companions.

When Rae's second husband died of a heart attack, she felt completely abandoned and that her life was finished. Not only was she mourning all her dead, she was also in a deep depression and felt that life had nothing more for her. For a week, while her remaining son was staying with her before he returned to Chicago, she stayed in her apartment and showed very little interest in anything. She was losing weight, becoming weaker, and was in her Dying Time. She was fading out of life and had already said good-bye to it.

The day before he had to leave, the son asked her to go downstairs to the pool area with him for a little while. She resisted for a time and then, as it seemed to her to be too much trouble to argue, she agreed. In the pool area he led her to a secluded place where there were two chairs, sat down with her, and said, "You see those women over there, sitting in the sun, reading magazines and talking about television programs and where to go for dinner? You have three choices as to what to do with your life, and which you choose is completely up to you.

You can, tomorrow or the next day, join them and be one of the crowd again. If you do, in a month you will wish even more than now that you were dead and in six months you will be dead. Or you can stay upstairs in your apartment and the same thing will be true. Except maybe a bit faster. Or you can realize something. This is the first time in your life that *no one* is making demands on you or depending on you to prepare meals for them and sew their clothes. All your life you have been taking care of others and now there are no others, there is only you. You have forty years of expertise in helping children to grow up and to find the work and way of life they needed. Now the only one to apply that expertise to is yourself, and you need it as much or more than they did. You are intelligent and able and have never found out what skills and abilities you have beyond home-making, and this is your last chance. You have a choice. What you decide will determine whether you have a miserable time and a bitter, empty death or whether you begin to find and enjoy your own life for the first time." As he delivered this strong speech, whose tone was far different from his usual way of relating to her, Rae looked at him with a startled and frightened expression. After he left the next day, she spent several days in her apartment. Then she looked up the numbers of a half-dozen social and charitable agencies in the telephone book, called them, and made appointments to meet with the director of volunteers. She interviewed them and found out what the organizations did and, in a few weeks, settled on a fund-raising organization for a hospital. Rae started by stuffing envelopes and in a year was directing the volunteers herself. At the end of three years, she was the (unpaid, but official) Executive Director of the organization and had also started the first real love affair of her life. For the next ten years she worked at least five days and several evenings a week with the organization.

Before her second husband had died, Rae had had a number of heart attacks and for the previous few years had been in an intensive care unit on the average of once a year. After she started working, these hospitalizations diminished in frequency so that she only had two within the next twelve years. Finally, at eighty-six, she suffered a very severe heart attack that killed her. Her last words to her son were "For the past ten years, I have loved my life."

I have written elsewhere in this book of the necessity for the therapist to have another approach to what it means to be human and in the human condition than that presented in the textbooks of psychiatry and psychology. This is particularly true of the therapist who works with people in the dying mode. What is in the textbooks is simply too narrow and sterile to deal with the great events of life such as leaving it. Whether one is a specialist in poetry, music, art, history, philosophy, or theology, the therapist needs to be aware of what the greatest minds of the human race have learned and communicated about the human condition long before there were these textbooks. My own approach is through poetry and I have, in this chapter and elsewhere in this book, given a few examples of the insights and statements of the English poets and, perhaps, how they can be useful in our understanding and in our work with patients.

In the need to complete our life before we leave it, very often people make a journey, either physically or in the mind, to their roots—whether to childhood places or to places and people who have been most central to our later lives. Often there is the need, in our integration process, to revisit and reexperience, as we are now, what shaped us and was so important to us.

In the beautiful movie *The Trip to Bountiful,* the actress Geraldine Page plays an old woman, living in an alien environment, coming toward her death, wanting desperately to visit again the town of Bountiful where she grew up. The town is abandoned now, the last person in it died by the time she gets there. After a difficult journey, made in the face of strong opposition of everyone else, she arrives and spends a few hours just looking at and reexperiencing the birds and the trees of her youth. She must then return to the hated city where she lives, but she goes now in peace. She has completed her death work. We know she will soon die and that this is no longer a cause for regret. She has completed her life. It is now a coherent whole.

Richard Cantwell, in Hemingway's *Across the River and into the Trees,* is also doing his death work. Conscious that he is going to die very soon, he reviews his life and realizes that he has attained the only real goal in his life—to be a General Officer in the United States Army. He consciously says good-bye to the two things he now loves the most, his girl and the city of Venice. Cantwell has come back to Venice to die because this is the place that meant the most to him during his life and where he would choose to live if he could. He looks at it for the last time, reexperiences and consciously says good-bye to everything that has made life meaningful for him. Then he goes over his entire life once more, pulling it together, feeling the pattern and meaning of it, and dies sadly but without regret or bitterness.

These are two cases from literature where the death work has been well done. In others an attempt was made and failed, where the person had no help or not enough inner resources or understanding of what the process was. I could show that these deaths are very different, torn by bitterness, anger, and regrets. Tolstoi's Ivan Ilyich would be one of these. Or the case of George Bowling from Orwell's *Coming Up for Air.* (Although Bowling does not die in the book, his end is foredoomed and clear.)

Some people do their death work by visiting in the flesh. After a heart attack, I felt a great need to visit the College of William and Mary where I, to a large degree, found myself as an adult and where I found many of the springs of enjoyment and meaning for my whole life. Going back to the psychology department there where I first found intellectual enjoyment and then being able to experience once more the trees and walks where I first grew up had deep meaning for me and brought a new peace to my life.

Others make the trip to Bountiful—the journey to the past to reintegrate it with the present so as to comprehend and experience the harmony and symphony of our lives—in other ways. In May Sarton's beautiful and important novel, *A Reckoning*, the protagonist Laura Spelman, bedridden and dying, brings to her bedside the most important person in her life and loving, a person from whom she has long been separated and who is now an eon and an ocean away. Together they talk and are with each other, and thus she completes her life. She dies in peace.

Some, like the woman Jung worked with, do it with inner exploration, either alone or with the aid of a friend, comrade, and/or psychotherapist. The journey can be made perhaps most effectively this way. Certainly in many deaths it is the only possible way. The places of the past cannot be visited physically either because they no longer exist, or more often, the person cannot leave the bed. The other people of importance may also not be able to come. But the journey can be made in the mind and the full integration made there. In Emily Dickinson's words:

> To make a prairie it takes one clover and a bee,
> And revery.
> The revery alone will do
> If bees are few.

No. 1775

Again, the importance of this final integration for a dying person cannot be overestimated. Without it the person's life is like a symphony without the last movement, the part in which all the previous themes are alloyed together in the triumphant finale.

There are some individuals who will reject the idea of working with a therapist during the Dying Time. Some prefer to die in the style in which they have lived and this may include people who have been very private in their feelings all their life. Others view not discussing their feelings as a way of maintaining their dignity. Among the other reasons are those people who prefer to die with their illusions intact rather than to explore them and possibly have to give them up.

One patient at the beginning of the fifth session we had (she was in the hospital with a metastasized breast cancer) told me that she did not wish to work further with me:

> I: I understand what you want and it is clearly your choice whether or not we go on. But there is one thing I would like to ask you. Not in order to argue with you or to try to change your mind. I must have done or said something stupid or hurtful. If I know what it is, then I won't do it again and hurt someone else as badly as I've obviously hurt you.
>
> PATIENT: No, it was nothing you did or said. It's just that I can see where we are going. If I continue to work with you, I will have to look at my marriage. And if I look at it, I'll lose it, and if it's a choice between my marriage and my life, I'd rather lose my life.

We parted amiably on this note. I dropped into her room from time to time and we remained friends until she died. She had made a conscious choice to maintain what she knew was an illusion and I could only accept and respect her choice and wish her well.

———

Jung, I believe, first advanced the concept that those of us who are fortunate as we go through life have a second adolescence. This generally occurs, if it does, between forty and sixty. In this developmental opportunity, we change our primary orientation from concern with the opinions of others to concern with the growth and becoming of our own being. Many do not pass through this stage. Others essay it and fail, usually then becoming more rigidly and concretely what they were before the attempt. Anyone with long hospital or hospice experience will have observed the difference in Dying Times between those who have passed this developmental stage and those who have not. Those who have made this shift come to their deaths with much less bitterness, regret, and despair. They have much less need of a psychotherapist; they are their own accepted and known comrade on the journey.

The Dying Time is the last chance to have the second adolescence. Often it can be completed now even though it may have been tried and failed many years previously. The basic goal and work of the psychotherapist during the Dying Time is defining and helping the patient with this task.

It is important to be aware of the fact that during their Dying Time, very often in the modern hospital, patients are hardly ever *touched.* I do not mean here that they do not receive basic medical care and are not turned over and bathed when necessary. Rather they are simply not touched in a caring, loving manner. Tolstoi's Ivan Ilyich received more comfort from the peasant Gerasim, who touched and held him during the last days, than he did from anyone else. In modern hospitals, nurses are often kept so busy doing things *for* patients, entering notes on the computer and keeping up charts, that they have very little time to be with patients or to touch them.

Some time ago I saw a man with lung cancer who was dying at home. His wife, who loved him deeply and was greatly hurt by what was going on, was so busy seeking after new treatment possibilities, consulting with doctors, nutritionists, and so on, and preparing an elaborate diet that she had neither the time or energy to be with him nor to touch him. An old Hungarian woman who was doing the physical housework kept coming over to him from time to time and would raise him up so she could fluff his pillows, straighten the sheets, support him with her arm while he drank some water, and so forth. I could see how comforting this was to him and how much he needed the physical contact and touch. Those who are with dying people should be aware that often people in this stage of life are on a touch-deficiency diet, and they should not be ashamed to help fill this need. For make no mistake, to be touched is a physiological and neurological as well as a psychological need. It relates strongly to patients' abilities to use the resources of their immune system as well as to be relaxed and comforted.

———————— ▬ ————————

I have written that one of the goals of the therapist working with the person who is in the dying mode is to help achieve a transcendent death as often as possible. This refers to a way of dying that everyone with long experience in a hospital has seen a number of times. Just before death—usually between one half hour and forty-eight hours before—the patient undergoes what is clearly a major personality change. This is not a change in any pathological sense, but rather the reverse. The word most usually used to describe the new state is *serene*. The person becomes serene and calm, and is obviously peaceful. He or she is clearly lucid and completely aware of everything going on around him or her, including the approaching death. The need for pain-reduction medication either disappears completely or is very much reduced. It is obviously not a change due to the drugs or body-breakdown products that sometimes cause negative personality changes in the very ill.

When the person is asked why he or she has changed, the person is unable to explain and often seems pitying of those who do not understand and therefore must ask. The most frequent reply is some variation of Louis Armstrong's famous answer when asked what jazz was. He said, "If you have to ask, you won't understand the answer."

Shakespeare commented on this (as have many other great writers): "How often when men are about to die have they been merry. What their keepers call 'a lightening before death.'" And indeed the word *merry* often seems applicable.

Various observers have also reported the acquiring of paranormal information at this time—as if telepathy were more common during a transcendent death.

No one has ever reported on the frequency of this phenomenon. My own (very rough!) estimate is that it occurs in one of fifteen or twenty patients who die slowly (not suddenly in a car accident, for example) and in a hospital. The percentage may be lower, however. In patients with whom I have worked and who have come to peace with their own lives, found and accepted its pattern, the percentage is very much higher—over 50 percent.

The meaning and causes of this phenomenon are far from clear. It appears, however, to be a valid goal to work toward when trying to help people in the dying mode. Certainly the surviving family seems to benefit from a death of this sort.

I suspect that there are also other ways, perhaps relevant for other cultures, for working toward helping the patient achieve transcendent death. The Tibetan tradition of having the family gather around the bedside of the dying person and chant a two-line verse over and over again may be this sort of attempt. The verse goes: "Nothing to hold to,/Nothing to do."

The basic key to working with people in their Dying Time is the oldest ethical rule of the western World: Do as you would be done by. This is the touchstone. How do you wish to be treated when you will be in your Dying Time? This, of course, is the touchstone for all good human relationships. It should not need to be stated here, but it does. It needs stating simply because we get so uptight when working with the dying, so self-conscious and artificial about our relationships, so complicated as to what we do, so driven by theories rather than by the basic rules of relating, that we forget this most elementary fact.

9

MEDITATION FOR CHANGE AND GROWTH

All through human history, there have been individuals who wanted the best of themselves and for themselves: they wanted to find a way to work in order to grow closer to their potential. Over and over again, in all the cultures of which we have record, they have invented a series of techniques that would enable them to work at this process. Curiously enough, these techniques, whether invented in India or Greece in the sixth century B.C., in second-century A.D. Japan, in the fifth to the fifteenth centuries in the Syrian and Jordanian deserts, in the medieval monasteries, in thirteenth-century Spain, or in Poland and Russia in the seventeenth and eighteenth centuries, or in many other times and places, were almost the same. They vary much more in detail than in essence. We call these techniques *meditations.*

The basic purpose of meditation is to help us recover something that we dimly perceive we once had and have lost: a spontaneity, an ability to be doing whatever we are doing with a whole heart and a full attention, a zest and startle at a sunset or a flower or a thought, an openness to new experience. We know that although we once had these things and have them no more, that they are still a part of our potential. Once we were a part of all reality; now we are only a part of a narrow segment including that which is within our skin and perhaps our family. Something within us yearns for wider vistas and broader skies. When we hear that that wise old psychologist Max Wertheimer defined an adult as "a deteriorated child," we smile with a sad recognition. When the meditator and mystic Louis de St. Martin was asked why he meditated so much and so long, he replied, "Because we are all in a widowed state and it is our task to remarry." The best single answer I have ever heard as to why someone meditated was by one professional scientist who said, "Because it's like coming home!"

Meditation, if worked at seriously and over a period of time, is a technique for growth and for integrating and nourishing the personality for future growth and change. It may be useful to compare it with psychotherapy—the other great gardening technique we humans have invented.

Both are serious methods. Both take a long time and hard work. (*There is no free lunch.*) Both are full of traps and false paths. Both are still primitive art forms, and we have a lot more to learn about them. The next major advance in this field may well be a synthesis that combines the best of both.

For our purposes there are, it seems to me, four separate types of meditation; actually four meanings of the word in common use today.

1. Listening to and following with our mind a speaker or a tape on a subject designed to relax us or to bring a high, wise, or good idea into our consciousness. We relax and follow this voice and often feel more relaxed, quieter, in less pain; more able to bear the pain we have; or more elevated and better for the meditation.

2. A second form is setting our mind a task, such as repeating one phrase (a *mantra*) over and over, and then relaxing and letting our minds go free. Whenever there is a blank in the stream of consciousness we repeat the phrase. This is a gentle, relaxing form of meditation and generally we feel better after it than we did before. It is most widely taught in the West by the school known as Transcendental Meditation.

3. In the third form, we actively work to visualize parts of the body (as cancer cells), in a symbol (such as small boxes of poisonous substances), and the healing forces of the body in another (such as small derricks). We then spend a planned amount of time each day visualizing the positive forces getting the negative elements out of the body. This method as a therapy for cancer was originated and most widely taught by Carl Simonton and Stephanie Simonton-Atchley and people they have trained. It has been most fully developed by Frank Lawlis and Jeanne Achterberg in their work and their books.

4. In the fourth method, an approach that is closest to the original and "classical" meaning of meditation, we work very actively to learn to do one thing at a time with our minds and to bring our minds more under our control. It is most analogous to the active work in a gymnasium and its purpose is to tune and train the mind as an athlete tunes and trains the body. Thus, if we choose the mantra method of repeating one phrase over and over again, we would, for the planned period of time, try very hard to do nothing else but that. We would strive to be as alert and awake as possible and be doing nothing else but repeating the phrase. Or if we choose another form of this method, to be doing nothing else but counting our breaths, looking at a seashell, or something like that.

In this "classical" method, we work to bring our total personality into a smooth-functioning whole so that it may be more efficient in accomplishing our purposes—so that we may be better at what we want to do and better at deciding what our goals are. Plato wrote that the mind of an adult is like a ship on which the crew have made a mutiny and locked the captain and the navigator down below in the cabin. There is a great feeling of freedom—as we ordinarily have with our minds—but, said Plato, this is an illusion. There is no freedom for all the parts of the mind to choose a goal, a harbor to go to, or if one is chosen, to navigate toward it. All the parts of the mind operate in an autonomous, free manner, and there is no unity. The task of an adult, Plato continued, is to quell the mutiny, to bring the captain and navigator up from below, and give them command so that a goal can be chosen and we can work our way toward it with a full crew, with all the parts of our being cooperating. This is the goal and rationale of classical meditation.

This type of meditation has two main thrusts. First, there is the tuning and training of the personality by trying to do one thing at a time, to bring one's consciousness more under one's control. Put this another way: to integrate the mind and personality so that we function more as a coherent whole, instead of as a collection of disparate parts.

The second thrust is to develop an attitude toward the self that can serve as a nourishment for further growth. We are, in this work, constantly prey to distractions, no matter how advanced we are or how much we have worked at it. Everyone's mind constantly wanders, be he or she novice or long-experienced teacher. Of major importance is how we bring ourself back to the work from these distractions. We learn to do this in a loving and supportive manner rather than in a self-condemnatory and self-accusative one. Meditating over a period of time builds up a positive attitude toward the self, a loving-but-demanding-the-best attitude that is an excellent soil for future growth.

This is not the place to go into real detail about the four types of meditation. Excellent books and teachers are available, and I refer to some of these in the Resource Directory. I will, however, make a few comments on them here.

1. All four kinds of meditation have real value. The first two, listening to a tape or speaker and giving oneself some time off from the problems of the world and everyday life to gently run a phrase through the mind, are excellent for relaxing and resting the total organism. They are the equivalent of using a hot whirlpool and a steam room, and having a good massage. They are certainly good for you and make you feel better. They help us to continue to deal with the problems and tasks we face, and often they enable us to make better rather than worse choices as to the paths of action we will take. For real *change*, however— if, for example, you wish to develop your muscles—active work is needed. There is, to put it simply and brutally, no easy way to change. If you wish to develop your body and change it, you will have to work at jogging, lifting weights, or the hard games of one sport or another that make you sweat and get tired. Both approaches are good for you. Only the second two, the ones with hard work in them, however, will change you.

Although this sounds rather Puritan, we have known this for a very long time. Not Jesus, Buddha, or Socrates, not Freud, Jung, or Adler, ever said that real change was easy or could be done without long, hard work. We have learned this truth, to our sadness and pain, from the thousands of years of experience of the esoteric schools and from a hundred years of experience with dynamic psychotherapy. As a matter of fact, we now use it as a test for teachers and gurus. If someone promises you real change in a short period of time (the odd couple of weekends, for example) or without major work on your part, this person is a charlatan. (Try asking these "wonderful" teachers what they know that none of the abovementioned teachers knew!)

2. Active visualization and classical meditation call for long and disciplined work. The visualization method is based on the idea that different parts of the personality use different *kinds* of language. If I wished to communicate with an Australian Bushman, whose language is entirely different from mine, I would use cartoon drawings—some sort of stick figures. This is the best way of communicating across language groups. Because the self-healing mechanisms are related to the personality at very "deep" levels, at levels that use a different kind of language from that used at conscious levels, we use cartoon-type figure symbols. Further, because communication of this kind is so difficult and chancy, we repeat the message over and over again in order (to use modern technical jargon) to push as much "signal" as we can through the "noise." The purpose of this form of meditation is to stimulate the person's own self-healing abilities and bring them to the aid of the medical protocol. For those patients for whom it "feels reasonable," it is often an excellent adjunct to the medical therapeutic program.

3. The "learn-to-work-at-being-able-to-do-one-thing-at-a-time" method also calls for long work. It is the equivalent, in some ways, of going to the gymnasium and lifting weights or using Nautilus machines. Very slowly our muscles develop, parts of us become larger, and parts of us become smaller as we get closer to our heart's desire. No one would expect us to really improve our figures in one or a few sessions, but we do change over time. Cardinal Newman wrote: "There is no such thing as a sudden enlightenment. There is, however, the sudden realization as to how much you have changed through long, hard work."

4. In both methods it is possible to work alone, in a group, or with a teacher. If you wish to work alone, or if circumstances make this necessary, there are excellent books to guide you. A number of these are listed in the Resource Directory.

If you work with a group, the most important thing to watch out for is competition. Psychological and spiritual growth is not like a ladder with one person ahead of another and the next person following behind. It is like a broad landscape with as many individual paths through it as there are people. Experiences on the road that one person has may never happen, or need to happen, to another. When working with a group you must realize that you are there to help each other on your unique and individual paths, not to compete with each other.

If you work with a teacher, remember that a second-rate teacher is worse than none. Ask yourself what kind of a human being this is: Does he or she have the kind of relationships with the self, others, and the world-at-large that you admire? After all, this person is saying to you "My knowledge of a system of growth enables me to help you grow toward where you want to be." Therefore, the system should have worked with the guru, or it is all a pretense. Further, does the teacher treat you as an individual? Does he or she say, "Let us find *your* dreams, celebrate them and help you on *your* individual path"? If, on the contrary, you are treated in a standardized way, leave unless you wish to become a standardized product. (And if this *is* something you wish, then I suggest you explore the desire to crush your own individuality. A good psychiatrist might help here!)

5. This brings up a crucial point about *all* meditational programs. In spite of the conflicting claims of so many teachers and schools, there is no one right way to meditate. There is a best way for each person at this particular stage of his or her development. The major reason that there are so many "failures" at meditation (people who start seriously, stop shortly thereafter, and never get back to it) is that so many schools say "There is one right way to meditate and by a curious coincidence it is the particular way we espouse!"

It is perfectly legitimate, and often important, for each person to try to learn how to work with a variety of techniques. Very often we cannot know if a meditation method is right for us until we try it, taste it, and work with it a bit. But, after this, a meditation program should be individually designed for you at your particular stage of your development. Work of this sort is not a suit you can take off the rack, no matter how fashionable it is at the moment. It should be individually hand-tailored for you. While one off the rack *may* fit you, the chances are against it. Anyone who says that he or she knows the right way for everyone to meditate has a great deal to learn about human beings. And it is particularly unhelpful, and can be harmful, to anyone with cancer.

6. Don't expect to achieve any final state. There is no such thing. Or, as Gertrude Stein put it: "When you get there you find there is no there there!" We work at our own growth in

order to move further along our path toward being at home with ourselves, with others, and with the universe. But the path is endless and there are always further vistas and possibilities ahead. (And who would really have it otherwise?) With anything serious—such as the ability to love, to appreciate beauty, one's personal efficiency in dealing with life, to learn and new ideas about which to learn—there is no end, no bottom. If we are truly lucky, and if we work at it, then all our lives we remain in a living room and do not move into a waiting room.

Meditation is one of the great paths that the human race has developed to further the growth of individuals and to help us move closer to our potential. It is a method of helping us grow and change and, as an adjunctive method in the treatment of cancer, can be of very great value.*

Charles, in his late forties, was generally regarded as a successful man. He was a writer and his novels had a good commercial success. They followed a formula. His readers knew pretty much what to expect and faithfully bought both hardcover and paperback editions. He was married and had a large house in the suburbs. His wife worked as a junior executive in a printing company.

They decided to adopt a child and began the usual long procedures. During the waiting time, Charles developed some symptoms and abdominal pain and went for a complete medical checkup. One Wednesday morning he received two communications. The first was a letter from the adoption agency saying that they now had a child for the couple. The second

*The ideas in this chapter are meant only as an overview. For greater detail, see my own How to Meditate or the other books listed in the Resource Directory.

was a telephone call from his physician stating that he had pancreatic cancer.

The medical workup resulted in a very poor prognosis. Radiation was not indicated, and the chemotherapy protocols available offered little hope. Charles decided to try one of them in spite of this—and of its generally distressing side effects— began it, and some two months later came to me for advice in setting up a meditation program.

He was not interested in psychotherapy. He had tried it twice in the past and found it uncomfortable and unpleasant. He told me he had always been a "loner," and preferred to work and try to solve problems by himself.

I explained to him that in order to design a meditation program specifically for him, I would have to know something about him and have a sense of who he was, how he had arrived at that point in his life, and what needed to be the main thrusts of the program. This approach appeared to make sense to the novelist in him, and over several hours of exploration a picture emerged.

Ever since early adulthood Charles had wanted to write "experimental" novels, to really explore new ways of viewing and describing the position of human beings in the twentieth century. He had always wanted the time to do this, to really devote himself to the task and to "become a real writer, not a hack!" But he had never been able to do it. When I asked why not, he said that he had to support a family, that he had obligations and needed to bring in a regular income.

I inquired, of course, who was in this family he had to support, as he sounded as if it were a large and heavy burden. He said that it was his wife. She was present at these interviews and had previously made it plain that she loved her work and that their tastes were fairly simple.

I responded that I thought that the reason he had given me for not really exploring and doing the work he said he wanted to was clearly nonsense. What, I asked, would his feelings be if he *did* have all the money he needed for the next three years and would be free, completely free, of all financial obligations and could devote himself fully to writing the kind of book he said he wanted so much to do? I asked him to imagine that situation and see how he felt.

Charles leaned back and thought for a long few minutes. Then he said, "I feel *terrified*. Suppose I found out that I was barren inside—that I really did not have what it takes to become a writer!"

This, he knew, was the real problem. The risk was just too great to take. He could bear anything else, any loss or pain or illness, but he could not cope with learning that he could not be a writer after giving it a full try. He had spent his life evading the critical test, blaming financial problems that did not exist.

The three of us talked about the situation for an hour. The couple could live comfortably for several years on the wife's income and their savings. In addition, if they sold their large house—which neither of them wanted, as both preferred their city condominium—they would be, in the wife's words, "very well off."

I pointed out to Charles that he now faced the situation he had most wanted and had fled from all his life. He had the opportunity, and it was now or possibly never, to face his worst fear. He talked about how terrifying it was and said that as long as he avoided the test, he could always believe that "if I had really tried, I could have done it." He said, "I could play Russian roulette with my body, but this is playing it with my soul, and *that* I'm too terrified to do."

The other factor that emerged in our discussion was how he really felt about the adoption procedures. Charles had known that a child was due to be available for them in the near future, and he had been in absolute despair about it. So long as he had no children, there were no real financial obligations to keep him from doing the writing experiment. His fantasy obligations kept him from doing this, but he somewhere knew that they were just fantasies. Some day, he felt, he would give them up and try! But with a child, he knew he never would. He had wanted a child to reinforce his fantasy that it was impossible for him to make the attempt. Really having one, however, meant the end of all hope; for him it permanently closed the door.

We set up a meditation program in terms of who he was—

as we could understand him—and the problems that needed to be faced and solved.

The first step in designing such a program is to determine what is "practical." I myself might wish that I were the kind of person who meditates an hour a day, but I am not. It is, therefore, a mistake to set up a program of this length because I simply will not do it. With the best intentions in the world, by the end of the first week I will begin to skimp and eventually to skip sessions until the whole program falls by the wayside. It is far better to acknowledge that I am a person who will, with full effort, meditate for half an hour a day, and set up a program of this length.

For Charles, a program of seventy-five minutes a day seemed acceptable. We talked about the wide range of kinds of meditation available and the kinds of effects they tended to have. We decided that the time would be divided into three twenty-minute periods with a five-minute period of nonagenda pause in between each of them and after the end of the last. During these five-minute pauses, he would just let himself be where he was and not attempt to exert any control on his mind.

The first meditation in the series was a visualization of the Simonton type. Of the many variations of this available, Charles chose, as feeling most *simpático*, to spend the twenty minutes visualizing his body as a harmonious, "flowing" whole in which all parts were "flowingly" interconnected to all the others and where nothing was extra or disturbed the total harmony. This "perfect working and relating" of the whole body would actively absorb or extrude nonharmonious aspects, such as the cancer.

The second meditation he chose was of the "classical" kind. In it, he would strive to be as awake and aware as possible and to be doing nothing but counting the exhalations of his own breath. This meditation of the "outer way" tends to, among other things, have positive effects on a person's feelings about his or her ability to cope with inner and outer events.

The third meditation he chose was of the "inner way," sometimes known as that of "the thousand-petaled lotus." In it, Charles chose one word or concept and, in a very highly structured way, explored his own associations to it. Among other effects, it tends to make us feel more at home with our inner life.

Charles felt that this program sounded relevant to him and promised himself to follow it rigorously and without exception (The rule is that you do it every day that there are no firemen and firehoses in the house!) for six weeks. At the end of that time, he would reconsider and decide if he wished to continue this route, if he wished to continue meditating the same length of time, and if he wished to continue to use the same meditations.

We talked about specific techniques and problems in meditating. Charles and I met several times in the next few weeks to discuss his program. At the end of six weeks, he decided to continue for another period of equal length, and then for a third. At the end of that time he changed two of the specific meditations for new ones. He continued to work in six-week programs, sometimes making changes at the end and sometimes not.

After about four months he decided one day that he was "ready." He was not aware of anything specific that had changed in him but felt that, frightened as he was, he could go ahead. He told his literary agent that he was taking some time off from his "regular" writing and was going to try some ideas he had had for a long time.

It was a hard and painful time. Charles had periods of depression and of anxiety. More and more, however, as the weeks went by, he became excited and involved in what he was doing. He told me that it was the hardest, most frustrating, and most rewarding time he had ever lived through. He said he felt more alive than he ever had before. Presently he was working on a series of vignettes and then these began to weave into a novel. It was completely different from anything he had ever written. He alternated between thinking it was very bad and very good. One day he told me it had passed a watershed—he felt the characters were now living the story and he was just recording it.

Soon the novel was finished and although he was

"exhilarated" about it, Charles decided to put it aside and start another to refine his new approach. He told me: "It's good, and I know now that I *am* a writer, that I have what it takes. But I have a lot more work to do before it will be what I want it to be. But I'll get there."

His response to the chemotherapy protocol was better than had been expected, and the size of the tumor reduced a good deal. After a three-month rest, another course of chemotherapy was started, which resulted in some more shrinkage. As there were now no further symptoms (except from the therapy), it was decided to go on a watch-and-wait program. This continued for another nine months with no change.

At the end of that time Charles was returning from the theater one evening when his car was hit by another car driven by a woman who had no license and had epileptic attacks. He was very badly hurt with extensive damage to the brain. He lost the ability to speak or write and had great difficulty walking. Two months later the cancer started to grow very rapidly, and Charles died shortly thereafter.

The experimental novel he had finished has been read by a number of knowledgeable people in the field who responded very positively to it. It has been accepted for publication and will be out in the near future.

EPILOGUE

As I was sitting in my office finishing this last chapter, the telephone rang. The voice at the other end said, "I am Raymondo Sanchez, do you remember me?" Immediately it all came back to my mind. Twenty-five years ago he and I had worked together. He had had cancer of the colon. For two and a half years we had seen each other nearly every week as he struggled to find out who he was and what was his own song to sing in life. At the end of that time, he knew that he wanted to return to the small Mexican city where he had been born and grew up. He left New York and returned to work as a dentist in an office on the town square rather than one he had had on 42nd Street and Eighth Avenue. I remember the description he had written in a letter of the square with its fountain and palm trees and the evening hours when everyone "promenaded" and then sat for long talkative, cheerful hours in the cafés. And I remembered his statements about how good he felt and how much he enjoyed his life—and how much energy he had.

We had corresponded a few times, and then I had heard nothing for over twenty years. We talked on the telephone for nearly a half hour. He was retired, just passing through New York on his way to see children and grandchildren in Canada. It was wonderful catching up with an old friend. I can think of nothing that says more what this work is about, or more illustrates the value to me of what I have been doing all these years, than that unexpected telephone conversation with my friend Raymondo Sanchez.

RESOURCE DIRECTORY

RECOMMENDED BOOKS RELATING TO THE PSYCHOLOGICAL ASPECTS OF CANCER

Achterberg, J. *Imagery in Healing.* Boston: Shambala, 1985.

————, and Lawlis, F. *Imagery of Cancer.* Champaign, Ill.: Institute for Personality Testing, 1978. Both of Achterberg's books are very valuable on the use of imagery in mobilizing the cancer-defense mechanism.

Borysenko, J. *Minding the Body: Mending the Mind.* Reading, Mass.: Addison-Wesley, 1987.

Cousins, N. *Anatomy of an Illness.* New York: W. W. Norton, 1979.

Dreher, H. *Your Defense Against Cancer.* New York: Harper & Row, 1989.

Jackson, E. *Coping with the Crises of Your Life.* New York: Hawthorn, 1974.

————. *Understanding Your Grief.* Nashville: Abingdon Press, 1957.

LeShan, E. *Learning to Say Good-by When a Parent Dies.* New York: The Macmillan Company, 1976.

————. *When a Parent Is Very Sick.* New York: Atlantic Monthly Press, 1986.

LeShan, L. *The Mechanic and the Gardener: How to Use the Holistic Revolution in Medicine.* New York: Holt, Rinehart & Winston, 1982.

————. *You Can Fight for Your Life: Emotional Factors in the Treatment of Cancer.* New York: Evans, 1979. This is the first book published in the field of helping the person with cancer to use a psychological approach to bring self-healing abilities to the aid of the medical program. It complements this book.

Pelletier, K. *Holistic Medicine.* New York: Delta, 1979. An outstanding holistic physician presents the field. Highly recommended.

Sarton, M. *A Reckoning.* New York: W. W. Norton, 1978.

————. *Recovering.* New York: W. W. Norton, 1980. In these two books, an outstanding novelist explores the psychological situation of the person with cancer and the person recovering from illness. Recommended very strongly as deeply insightful.

Siegel, B. *Love, Medicine and Miracles.* New York: Harper & Row, 1987. The most widely read book in the field.

Simonton, O. C.; Simonton, S.; and Creighton, J. *Getting Well Again.* New York: Bantam, 1980. This book introduced the idea of using imagery to help cope with cancer.

RECOMMENDED BOOKS ON MEDITATION

LeShan, L. *How to Meditate.* Boston: Little, Brown, 1974; New York: Bantam, 1975.

Merton, T. *The Ascent to Truth.* New York: The Viking Press, 1951.

Naranjo, C., and Ornstein, P. *The Psychology of Meditation.* New York: The Viking Press, 1971.

Underhill, E. *Practical Mysticism.* London: P.J.M. Dent, 1914; Harmondsworth, England: Penguin, 1970. Probably the outstanding classic in the field. Eminently readable.

RECOMMENDED CANCER HELP ORGANIZATIONS

Cancer Care, 1180 Sixth Avenue, New York, NY 10036. 212-302-2400. An excellent organization with a very practical approach. Provides support and information for people with cancer and their families.

Commonweal, P. O. Box 316, Bolinas, CA 94924. 415-868-0790. An organization that gives excellent five-day seminars for people with cancer. It also has very good material on the nonmainline treatment methods, both adjunctive and alternative. Five-day seminars of the same sort for people with cancer and their immediate families, are also given at Wainright House, 260 Stuyvesant Avenue, Rye, NY 10580. 914-967-6080. These seminars give excellent suggestions on how to cope most effectively and richly with the illness.

Exceptional Cancer Patients, New Haven, CT. 203-865-8392.

Independent Citizens Research Foundation, Inc., P. O. Box 97, Ardsley, NY 10502. A highly responsible source of information about alternative methods of cancer treatment.

Cancer Counseling Inc., P. O. Box 980637, 2211 Norfolk, Suite 927, Houston, TX 77098-0637. 713-520-9873.

Many local societies are devoted to providing information, counseling, and support to cancer patients. Typical of the best of these are:

Life After Cancer, Asheville, NC
To Life, Charlotte, NC
Living Through Cancer, Albuquerque, NM

Special centers providing information and support regarding the holistic treatment of illness, including cancer, are rapidly springing up not only in the United States but all over the world. In Bristol, England, for example, The Cancer Help Centre (Clifton, Bristol, B58 4PG, Tel. 0272-743216) has achieved international recognition for the very high quality of its services.

RECOMMENDED MATERIALS FOR HEALTH PROFESSIONALS

There is now a very extensive and rapidly growing literature in the area of the psychological aspects of cancer, literature far too large to present here. The following publications are essential reading for psychotherapists and other health professionals.

Bahnson, C. B. "Stress and Cancer: State of the Art." *Psychosomatics* 27 (1980).

Baltrusch, H. J. F., and Walter, M. B. "Stress and Cancer: A Psychobiological Approach." *Current Advances* 2 (1988).

Booth, G. "Psychobiological Aspects of 'Spontaneous' Regression of Cancer." *Journal of the American Academy of Psychoanalysis* 3 (1973).

Grossarth-Matick, D. "Social Psychotherapy and Course of Cancer." *Psychotherapy and Psychosomatics* 33 (1980).

Kissen, D. M. "Psychosocial Factors, Personality and Lung Cancer in Men." *British Journal of Medical Psychology* 40 (1967).

Klopfer, B. "Psychological Variables in Human Cancer." *Journal of Projective Techniques* 21 (1957).

LeShan, L. "A Basic Psychological Orientation Apparently Associated with Neoplastic Disease." *Psychiatric Quarterly* (1961).

————. "An Emotional Life History Associated with Neoplastic Disease." *Annals of the New York Academy of Sciences* 125 (1966).

————. "Psychological States as Factors in the Development of Neoplastic Disease: A Critical Review." *Journal of the National Cancer Institute* 22 (1959).

————., and LeShan, E. "Psychotherapy and the Patient with a Limited Life Span." *Psychiatry* 24 (1961).

List, M. A., *Respectful Treatments.* Harper and Row. New York, 1977.

Pettingale, K. W.; Philithis, D.; and Greer, H. S. "The Biological Correlates of Psychological Response to Breast Cancer." *Journal of Psychosomatic Research* 25 (1981). This reports on part of the most important modern *prospective* study of the relationship of personality and survival time in persons with cancer.

"Psychosocial Aspects of Cancer: Reports of Two Conferences." *Annals of the New York Academy of Sciences* (January 21, 1966). *Annals of New York Academy of Sciences* (October 4, 1969).

Spiegel, D., Bloom, J. R., Kraemer, H. C. and Gottheil, E., "Effect of Psychosocial Treatment on Survival of Patients with Metastic Breast Cancer." *Lancet.* (October 14, 1989.)

Thomas, C., and Greenstreet, R. "Psychological Characteristics in Youth as Predictors of Five Disease States." *Johns Hopkins Medical Journal* 132 (1973). This is the first, and a major, modern prospective study of psychological factors and the appearance of cancer.

Tolstoi, L. *The Death of Ivan Ilyich.* New York: New American Library, 1960. Essential reading for anyone working in the cancer field.

Weinstock, C. "Recent Progress in Cancer Psychobiology and Psychiatry." *Journal of the American Society of Psychosomatic Medicine and Dentistry* 24 (1977).

Further, health professionals should be familiar with the work of:

European Working Group for Psychosomatic Cancer Research (EUPSYCA)
Chairman: Dr. H. J. F. Baltrusch
Bergstrasse 10
D-1900, Oldenburg, Federal Republic of Germany

By the year 2000, 2 out of 3 Americans could be illiterate.

It's true.

Today, 75 million adults...about one American in three, can't read adequately. And by the year 2000, U.S. News & World Report envisions an America with a literacy rate of only 30%.

Before that America comes to be, you can stop it...by joining the fight against illiteracy today.

Call the Coalition for Literacy at toll-free **1-800-228-8813** and volunteer.

Volunteer Against Illiteracy. The only degree you need is a degree of caring.